18

LIFE IS LONG!

KAREN
SALMANSOHN

LIFE IS LONG!

50+ WAYS TO HELP YOU LIVE A LITTLE BIT CLOSER TO FOREVER

ILLUSTRATIONS BY
SARAH FERONE

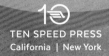

TEN SPEED PRESS
California | New York

CONTENTS

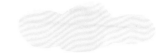

Acknowledgments

I'd love to thank my amazing editor on this book, Lisa Westmoreland. I consider Lisa my soul mate editor; she always brings out the best in me—and edits, polishes, and deletes the worst in me.

Next up, my awesome agent entourage who helped bring this life-boosting book to life! Big appreciation to Celeste Fine, Jaidree Braddix, Sarah Passick, and Anna Petkovich.

Next up I'd like to thank my favorite concierge doctor, Bruce Yaffe, MD, for helping to keep me healthy and thriving—and helping to vet this book so it's jam-packed with the best longevity tools.

I'd also love to share my appreciation for my brilliantly talented designer, Leona Chelsea Legarte, the awesomely gifted illustrator, Sarah Ferone, my crack marketing and publicity team, Daniel Wikey and Eleanor Thacher, and my amazing production manager, Serena Sigona.

Thank you, Fred DeVito, for cofounding EXHALE, my favorite workout destination, which helps keep me young in body and spirit.

Lastly, thank you to those who are making it worthwhile to live to one hundred-plus: Ari Salmansohn, Howard Schwartz, Shelly Lipton, Danielle Pashko, Kristine Carlson, Bonnie Winston, Kristy Lin, Michael John Hughes, Karen Giberson, Richard Kastleman, Michelle Spector, Ira Garr, Safije Alija, Dominique Misrahi, Denise Barry, Lisa Attea, Marcia Bronstein, Gloria Salmansohn, Eric Salmansohn, Lia Salmansohn, Ross Salmansohn, and many others—too many to list, but you know who you are!

Introduction

Want to live to one hundred—and feel thirty? Me too!

I'm a late-in-life mom, and I want to be around to dance at my son's wedding. With this in mind, I recently promised my son, Ari, that I'd do everything I can to live to one hundred.

Ari wanted me to live to two hundred, but I bargained him down to one hundred.

Ari accepted my counteroffer.

As a happiness and wellness expert, I've always been interested in living a healthy lifestyle. But after my vow to be a centenarian, I became particularly passionate about learning and practicing as many healthy habits as I could memorize and muster.*

It's because I'm fascinated with health and wellness that I studied to become a yoga and meditation teacher at the amazing ISHTA Yoga studio. In fact, I was never interested in teaching classes. I simply wanted to learn the science and logic behind why yoga and meditation are such health game changers—and how best to use these tools to win at the longevity game!

*Note: If you think genetics is the biggest predictor of how long you're gonna live, then you need to think again! A famous Danish twin study reported that only about 20 percent of how long the average person lives is predetermined by genetics.

I also began reading stacks of books and interviewing and immersing myself in the wisdom of a range of health experts, from Fred DeVito, cofounder and EVP of Exhale, to Dr. Mark Hyman, internationally recognized health leader, to Howard Friedman, the force of nature behind the Longevity Project—and then some.

I also spoke with my favorite concierge doctor, Bruce Yaffe, MD*, who's been my go-to personal physician for about twenty years. I'm not the only fan of Dr. Yaffe; for more than ten years *New York* magazine has named him a Best Doctor in NYC and a Best Doctor in the USA. Dr. Yaffe is very involved with groundbreaking research on longevity. He's active in the New York Stem Cell Foundation and passionate about research on whole genome sequencing, genetic predisposition, microbiomes, Nrf2s—all the cutting-edge longevity exploration currently going on around the globe.

Dr. Yaffe's focus as my physician is on preventive maintenance and keeping his patients healthy in five key categories: (1) mobility, (2) brain function, (3) heart/lung/cardiovascular health, (4) sensory function (hearing, vision, taste, smell), and (5) economic/monetary healthiness! Every time I see Dr. Yaffe he reminds me to think preventively about my health—not only about how I eat but also how I shower, drive, and sleep. Thanks to Dr. Yaffe, I have a sturdy nonslip bath mat in my tub, nonslip rugs in my living room, a night-light on at bedtime, seat belts on in every car ride—and I always look out for cyclists when I exit cars. Dr. Yaffe warns, "I've seen far too many patients who take good care of their health by eating right and regularly exercising—then one day they aren't careful, they have an accident, and suddenly their quality of life is taken away from them!"

I also read up on the secrets of peppy people in the "Blue Zone"— geographic regions around the globe where folks are regularly known to live to ninety or even one hundred years old.

*I not only interviewed Dr. Yaffe, I also had him vet all the research and suggestions in this book!

What you hold in your hands is the handy, fast-paced, curated result of all the hours I put into researching the secrets of living both longer and younger. I wanted to snag two out of two. After all, I'm not simply interested in increasing my quantity of years on this planet; I also want to improve the *quality* of those years.

I've grouped the tips in this book into two buckets: body and mind. As it turns out, longevity is linked to not only physical health but also mental well-being! The first half of the book contains the body-focused tips (colored blue in the table of contents). The second half features the mind-focused tips (in a pretty teal color!).

Regardless of whatever your present age might be, I know the tools in this book will help you—because they've already helped me!* I definitely feel younger and more energetic. Friends, family, and coworkers also keep telling me that I don't look (or act) my age.

I even fooled my blood lab into believing I'm younger.

I had my blood tested recently. Dr. Yaffe joked with me: "Karen, you have the Harvard of blood tests for someone your age!"

Meaning? My blood doesn't look, feel, or act its age either.

*Reminder: Ask your doctor before undertaking any changes to your health regime, from trying a new supplement to testing out something like intermittent fasting.

I'd love to help your blood behave age-inappropriately as well. With this in mind, I'm excited to share all that I learned in my quest to live to one hundred plus!

After all, the more people who live to one hundred plus alongside me, the more people who will come to my one-hundredth birthday party. And I promise it will be a super fun bash.

Oh, and I'm not joking! I'm actually planning my one-hundredth birthday party now—for two researched reasons.

- I want to engage in *plan de vida* ("reason to live")—a common practice of peppy elders living in Nicoya, Costa Rica, a famed centenarian hot spot. In Nicoya, residents credit their longevity to living with a purpose. (Example: Looking forward to fun times with family and friends.)

- I want to positively embrace getting older. According to a study published in the *Journal of Personality and Social Psychology*, people who enjoy a happy attitude about aging lived more than seven years longer than those with negative attitudes about aging.

So I'm planning my one-hundredth birthday party—for real! And you are invited! Head on over to my website and sign up to be on the invite list at notsalmon.com/100bdaybash.

Although it's my birthday bash, I'll send you lots of gifts—long before my one-hundredth birthday—including free longevity videos and discounts on lots of longevity products.

And as always, I'd love for my books to be a two-way conversation. If you have a good longevity tip or an inspiring story about a special centenarian in your life, please write to me via my website, NotSalmon.com!

Here's to knowing you for a long, long time . . .

XO
Karen

If you want to read all the fascinating articles, studies, and quotation sources for yourself, visit notsalmon.com/life-is-long-endnotes. The sources are organized by topic for easy reading. Also, if any cool new research comes along, I'll be adding it there as well!

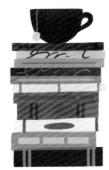

1

EAT LIKE AN IMMORTAL: PRACTICE "HARA HACHI BU"

There's a Blue Zone region in Japan called Okinawa, nicknamed "the land of the immortals"—because people often live to age one hundred.

One of their secrets is *hara hachi bu*—the practice of eating until you're only 80 percent full. It helps if the food you eat is unprocessed whole foods*, but simply learning to eat until you're 80 percent full can be life boosting.

Unfortunately, it's easy for anyone to overeat, because it takes about twenty minutes for the tummy to communicate to the brain just how full it is. And a lot of forkfuls can happen in twenty minutes!

THE SOLUTION?

- Chew slower.

- Make a conscious choice to eat smaller portions.

- Refuse second helpings.

- Excuse yourself to go to the restroom mid-meal so you have time to feel, for real, how full you are.

- Drink a tall glass of water thirty to sixty minutes before a meal.

*Some Okinawan fave cuisines are tofu, goya (bitter melon), and stir-fried veggies—with a special emphasis on sweet potatoes and taro roots!

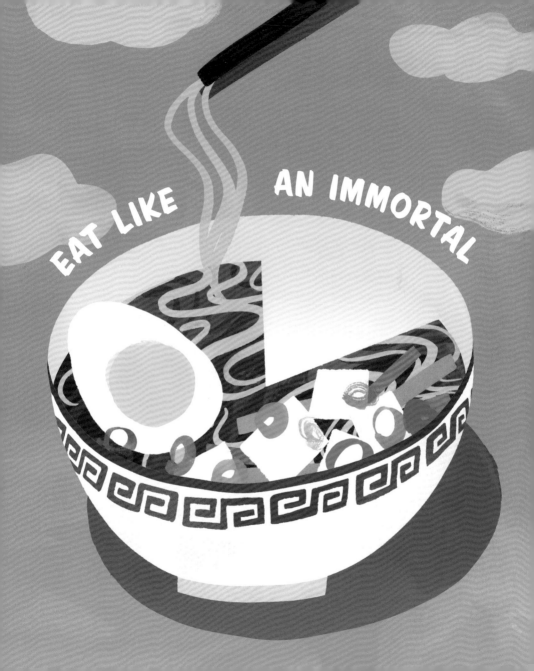

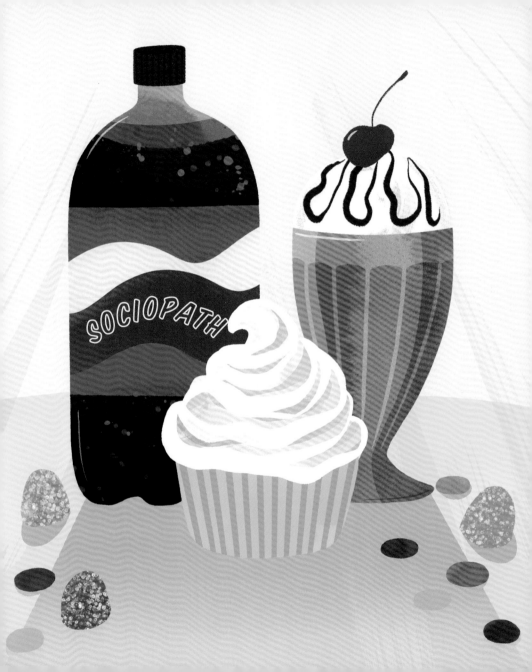

2

WARNING: SUGAR IS A SOCIOPATH!

Yes, sugar is super sweet.

But beware!

Sugar is a dangerous, two-faced sweetie—killing millions of people with heart disease, cancer, dementia, and type 2 diabetes.

"Sugar [is] the new cigarettes," says Dr. Mark Hyman, famed antisugar crusader and founder of the UltraWellness Center.

Dr. Hyman cites a Harvard study in which folks consumed either high-sugar milkshakes or low-sugar ones. The high-sugar shakes "spiked blood sugar and insulin and led to sugar cravings," says Dr. Hyman. "It lit up the addiction center in the brain like the sky on the Fourth of July. Think cocaine cookies, morphine muffins, or smack sodas!"

So how do you stop sugar addiction?

Danielle Pashko, a highly respected nutritionist and author, recommends the following:

- Get savvy about sugar's hiding places. Avoid processed foods, flavored yogurts, energy bars, and store-bought bread.

- Know sugar's aliases. Sugar goes by many names, like high-fructose corn syrup, sucrose, and maltose.

- Make room for magnesium. Sugar cravings may be more pronounced in people who don't get enough magnesium. So start eating more dark leafy greens, nuts, seeds, fish, and beans.

- Power up with cinnamon. It not only lowers blood sugar levels, but also reduces heart disease risk factors. So get sprinkling!

3

EAT SIT AND DIE

If you were asked to name a habit that's linked to heart disease, dementia, and even cancer, I bet sitting wouldn't be at the top of your list.

But lack of enough physical activity has been identified as the fourth-leading risk factor for death for people all around the world, according to the World Health Organization. Research shows that sitting eight to twelve hours or more a day increases your risk of developing type 2 diabetes by 90 percent—and has been linked to high blood pressure, obesity, and bad cholesterol.

Plus, prolonged sitting is a silent killer that's harmful not only physically, but also mentally. A major study from Boston University School of Medicine discovered that people who were couch potatoes in their thirties and forties were more likely to have smaller brains two decades later.

Basically, a sedentary lifestyle accelerates the aging process, speeding the rate at which the brain shrinks.

TWO WAYS TO STOP YOUR SITTY BEHAVIOR:

1. Motion is a health potion. Aim to get up every thirty minutes or so. Set a timer! Do a few jumping jacks or a simple set of stretches. Go get a glass of water. Get your blood flow going! Added bonus: When you take breaks away from your computer screen, you're doing your eyes a favor at the same time. Win-win.

2. Switch up the landscape. Who says work meetings have to be inside? Walk your talk, and do meetings circulating in a park. Bonus: A change in scenery often leads to a change in thinking.

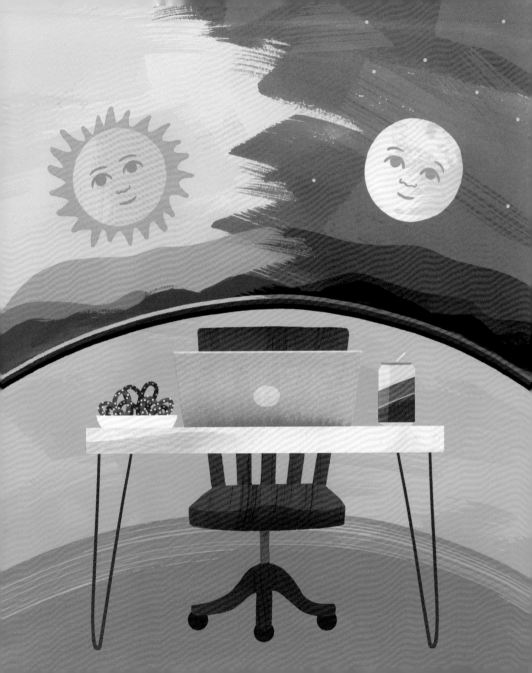

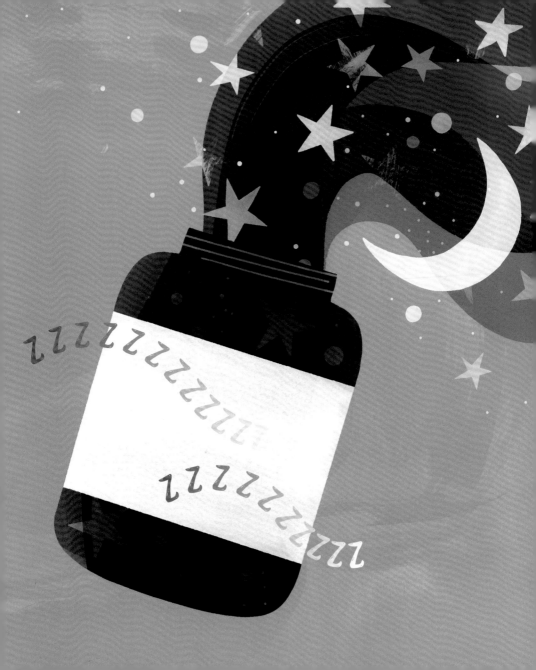

4

GET YOUR VITAMIN ZZZZZ'S

In 2002 Daniel Kripke, codirector of research at the Scripps Clinic Sleep Center, found that people who consistently sleep less than six and a half hours a night don't live as long as people who sleep seven to eight hours a night.

In 2012 a Penn State study also found a link: People who slept less than six hours a night were four times more likely to die than those who got a full eight hours.

Plus, the Cancer Treatment Centers of America reports that there are many studies linking lack of sleep with some of the top cancers in the United States: breast, prostate, and colorectal.

If you want more motivation to hit the hay earlier, consider the sleep habits of the many famed centenarians living in the Blue Zones. They report regularly getting a full, restful eight hours of sleep.

YOUR ASSIGNMENT:

- Try to go to bed at the same time and wake up at the same time. Your body will regulate to this cycle, and it will be easier to fall asleep and wake up energized.

- Resist caffeine after 3 p.m. (It has a twelve-hour lasting effect!)

- Don't watch TV or use your computer in bed. However, reading in bed is allowed—but only if you're reading this book! Just kidding! Seriously, according to researchers at the University of Sussex, reading is terrific at reducing stress levels, which can help you fall asleep.

- Stop eating at least three hours before bedtime. This will help you avoid acid reflux and sleep apnea.

5

LIVE MORE SEASONS
WITH SEASONINGS

Add these seasonings to your meals and smoothies—and you might just add more years to your life!

OREGANO

Oregano and its oil have four times as much antioxidant power as blueberries on a per-ounce basis! And one tablespoon of fresh oregano gives you the same antioxidant boost as a medium-size apple. Plus, the beta-caryophyllin in oregano oil helps reduce inflammation.

TURMERIC

Turmeric extract can lower your risk of heart attack by 56 percent, says a study in the *American Journal of Cardiology*. And turmeric can improve your cardiovascular health as much as aerobic exercise, according to a 2012 study in the *Nutrition Research Journal*. Crazy but true—thanks to its having a primary polyphenol called curcumin. Turmeric/curcumin is also reported to protect the brain, prevent inflammation, and help combat cancer.

CLOVES

Cloves tend to be used in the kitchen only seasonally (pumpkin pie, anyone?), but in research labs they're revered for having the highest ORAC (oxygen radical absorbance capacity) score of all spices. Meaning? They're the highest in antioxidants. Cloves are also effective for eliminating intestinal parasites, fungi, and bacteria.

GINGER

Ginger contains geraniol, recommended as a potent cancer fighter. Plus, ginger is an anti-inflammatory, known for being helpful for your heart and beneficial at preventing blood clots. It's recommended for boosting the immune system and touted as protecting against atherosclerosis.

tumeric

ginger

oregano

cloves

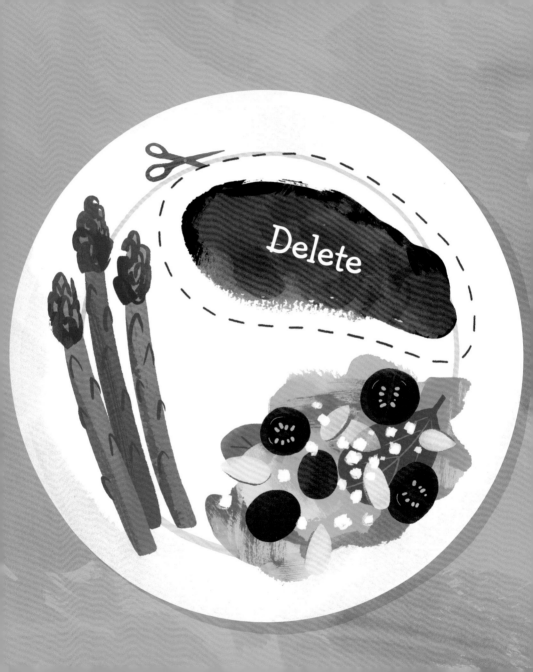

6

DELETE MEAT

Lower your meat consumption and lower your risk of death.

Says who? A report in the *American Journal of Clinical Nutrition*, which compared different studies to determine whether vegetarians live longer than devout meat devourers.

The meaty details: Reducing meat consumption can increase your life span by 3.6 years or more.

The reasoning? People who eat meat are more likely to have high cholesterol, which increases the chances of heart disease. Plus, according to a 2006 article in *Life Extension*, eating meat was also reported to increase the risk of certain cancers, such as colon cancer, as well as kidney stones and gallstones.

If you feel challenged to delete, start with red meat. It has more cholesterol and saturated fat than white meats.

HOW TO PLANT POWER YOUR BODY:

- Choose healthy veggies—legumes and roots and leaves, especially dark leafy greens—and low-sugar fruits; avocados; seeds such as chia, hemp, sunflower, and flax; nuts such as Brazil nuts, walnuts, cashews, and almonds; and ancient whole grains such as millet and quinoa.

- Buy local and organic whenever possible (because they're fresher and contain higher levels of antioxidants and less harmful chemicals)—or grow your own!

EXTRA VEGETARIAN POINTS: Don't just focus on more greens! Get your blue-greens, too—in the form of spirulina, a protein-rich superfood that contains all the essential amino acids and can be added directly to juice or water.

1

GET YOUR COFFEE BUZZ ON!

I love coffee. As it turns out, coffee loves me right back!

A Harvard study reports that moderate coffee drinking is linked to a 15-percent lower risk of premature mortality.

Meaning? In the past I've always lived for coffee. But now I can also live longer because of coffee!

Says who? Dr. Ming Ding, a Harvard researcher involved in a coffee study done on more than 208,000 men and women over a thirty-year period. He reported that those who drank three to five cups of caffeinated or decaffeinated coffee per day had a lower risk of death from type 2 diabetes, cardiovascular disease, neurological diseases such as Parkinson's disease—and even suicide.

Dr. Ming Ding explains: "It could be that certain compounds in coffee, such as chlorogenic acid, may help reduce insulin resistance and inflammation, which are associated with many diseases."

Another researcher, Dr. Walter Willett, has suggested that compounds in coffee—such as lignans, quinides, and magnesium—may help reduce insulin resistance and inflammation.

Researchers from Indiana University report that the caffeine in coffee may boost an enzyme (NMNAT2) in the brain that protects against dementia.

TWO WARNINGS:

- Coffee beans are one of the most notoriously sprayed crops. Try to buy certified organic.

- You can have too much of a good caffeine thing! Research also shows that consuming more than 400 milligrams of caffeine can interfere with sleep.

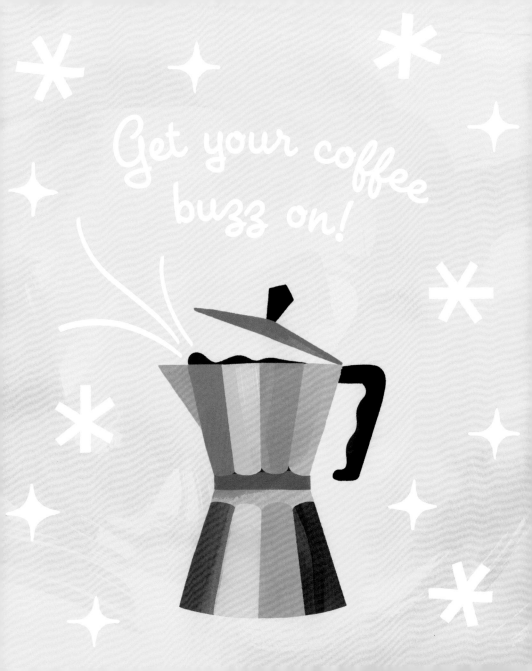

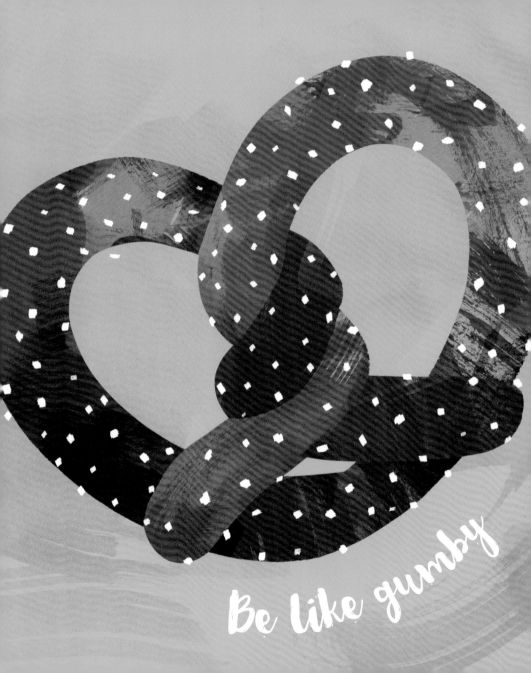

Be like gumby

BE LIKE GUMBY

You'll have to sit down for this longevity tool. Literally sit down. Try this.

Sit down on the floor, then get back up using as little support as possible—no hands!

How did you do?

A study in the *European Journal of Preventive Cardiology* reports that your level of ability to do this sitting-rising test can predict how long you're going to live.

The study looked at two thousand people ages fifty-one to eighty. They told the men and women not to worry about how fast they did the test, just simply focus on using as little support as they could.

The results?

A follow-up 6.3 years later found that 159 of the study subjects had died—and

of those, the majority had had the most trouble going from sitting to rising.

Researchers also found that if a subject's score was an eight to ten on the test (meaning greater ability to get up without support), they happily had a five to six times lower risk of death compared to those who scored a three or lower on the test.

IN SUMMARY: Yoga pants are not just something you put on to do errands. Wear them to a yoga class and work on your musculoskeletal fitness: your flexibility, balance, muscle strength, and coordination. Then do the sitting-rising test again and see how much better you do!

9

EAT FOODS WITHOUT A BARCODE

One of the biggest longevity tips—supported in study after study—and found in all the famed longevity Blue Zones: eat real, unpackaged, unprocessed foods!

Basically, if a food has a barcode on it, chances are it's less good for you than a version that does not.

With this in mind, I've pretty much cut processed and packaged foods out of my diet.

The willpower tool that helps me resist?

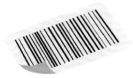

I REMIND MYSELF OF THE FOLLOWING MANTRAS:

- The longer a food's shelf life, the shorter my shelf life on this planet!

- Processed food is dead food—and I am what I eat!

- Eating fresh fruits and fresh veggies keeps my body fresher longer!

- If I don't recognize an ingredient, my body won't either!

- If I have trouble pronouncing the ingredients with my mouth, then I shouldn't put the food in my mouth. (Unless it's, say, quinoa or acai!)

- If the food has ingredients I would not stock in my kitchen pantry, then I shouldn't eat it.

- Being healthy is not just about counting the calories in my food—it's also about counting the chemicals in my food!

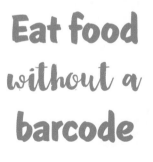

Eat food
without a
barcode

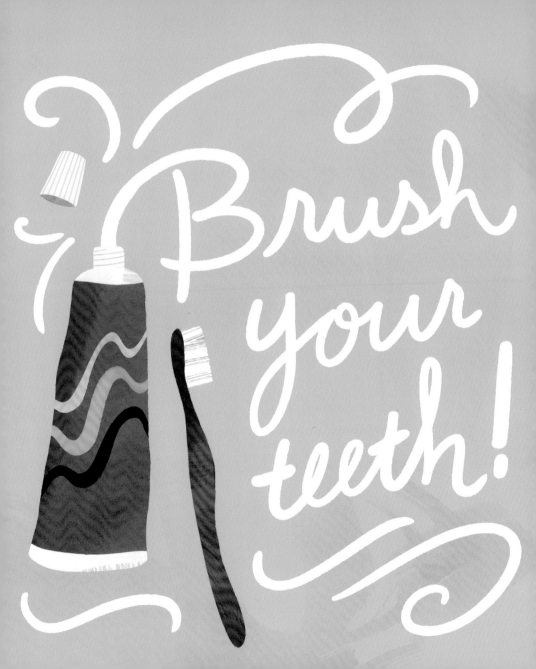

IF YOU DON'T WANT TO BITE THE DUST, BRUSH YOUR TEETH!

You're gonna want to brush up on these longevity facts: brushing your teeth regularly could reverse early signs of heart disease.

How the heck are your teeth connected to your heart? Via traveling oral bacteria!

The full story: Researchers at the University of Milan discovered that a specific bacteria in the mouth—*Porphyromonas gingivalis*—is a huge culprit in not only gum disease but also heart disease.

Dr. Mario Clerici, the study leader and an immunologist, said he was surprised to learn that something as simple as taking care of your gums could reverse lesions in the blood vessels that could lead to heart disease.

Dr. Clerici explains that the bacteria in the mouth trigger an immune response that increases the production of T lymphocytes, a vital part of the body's immune system. However, once the immune system starts to attack the bacteria, it moves on to the proteins in all the blood vessels and ultimately to the heart.

WHAT TO DO?

- Dr. Clerici's recommendation? Take good care of your teeth and gums, so you reduce both oral bacteria and the risk of atherosclerosis and cardiovascular disease.

- Aging expert Dr. Tom Perls agrees! He says flossing daily could add more than a year to your life.

- New York City oral surgeon Dr. Keith Lustman's sum-up? "Be true to your teeth—or they'll be false to you!"

11

LIVE A BERRY, BERRY LONG TIME

A teeny tiny blueberry holds a big secret to a long life—a powerful little something called "polyphenols."

Gobbling up lots of polyphenols has been reported to create a 30-percent reduction in incidence of mortality in older adults, according to consistent studies, including a 2013 multi-institutional report published in the *Journal of Nutrition*.

How does such a little-guy berry pack such a big longevity punch?

The polyphenols that blueberries are blessed with are known for their antioxidant, anti-inflammatory, and anticarcinogenic properties, protecting you from oxidative stress and cardiovascular disease.

Plus, polyphenols are big-time beneficial for blood pressure, insulin resistance, and something called lipid metabolism—which, loosely translated, means the ability to convert fats into energy.

Happily, you can be polyamorous about your polyphenol food sources—and not get them only from blueberries!

OTHER YUMMY SOURCES OF POLYPHENOLS: blackberries, dark chocolate, red wine, coffee, nuts, green tea, kale, spinach, and a variety of spices like ginger and cumin.

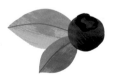

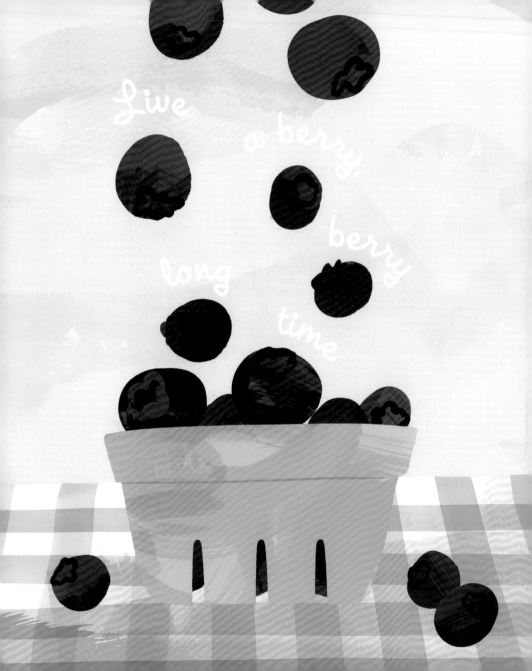

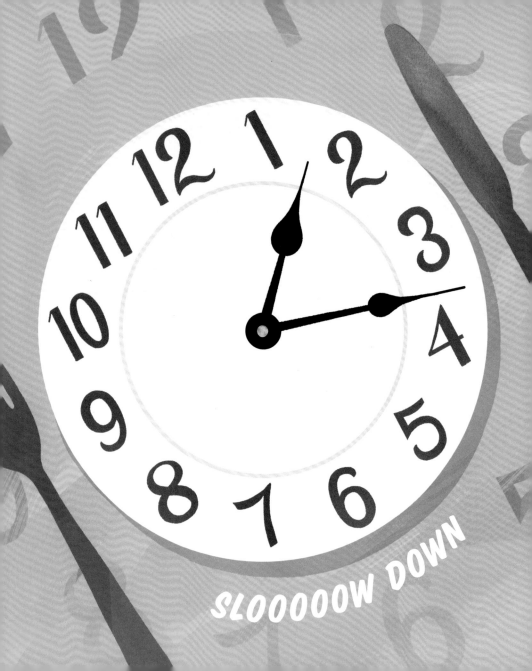

SLOOOOOW DOWN

12

TRY A FAST TO
SLOOOOOW DOWN AGING

An abundance of research suggests that intermittent brief fasting is an effective longevity tool.

Why? When you stop eating for ten to sixteen hours, you increase your mitochondrial energy efficiency, and your body burns fat as its energy source. This combo slows down aging and disease.

Basically, the mightier your mitochondria, the mightier your chances of living longer.

For this reason, intermittent fasting is now being widely touted for boosting health, metabolism, and weight loss— even over the once-popular "grazing" recommendation.

Surprising but true: A study published in *Cell Metabolism* reported that mice who continually grazed on food for one hundred days gained weight and

developed high cholesterol, high blood glucose, and liver damage. In contrast, mice who fasted for sixteen hours a day but ate the same total amount of food during nonfasting periods weighed less, stayed healthy, and performed better when exercising.

IF YOU'D LIKE TO TRY IT YOURSELF:

- Make sure your evening meal the night before contains a good amount of fats and protein to ensure stable blood sugar levels.

- Be sure to stay hydrated.

BONUS: The *American Journal of Clinical Nutrition* reports that intermittent fasting lowers LDL ("bad") cholesterol and triglycerides—but not HDL ("good") cholesterol.

13

GIVE YOURSELF AN OIL CHANGE

Not all oils are created equal—or evil.

Oil yourself up in the right ways and you can oil rig your health for better longevity odds.

The good fats found in the right oils can fuel your body, help you feel fuller faster, stimulate fat burning, even prevent and treat a range of diseases.

Studies show these good fats are also a helpful part of a ketogenic diet (low in carbs and high in fats from healthy oils and foods), shown to improve longevity odds and prevent diseases like Parkinson's, brain tumors, and diabetic kidney disease.

The ketogenic diet includes high-quality fats from healthy oils and foods—around 70 to 80 percent of your daily calories. Studies show these help with production of mitochondria, an important longevity factor. The ketones your body generates in response increase glutathione, a powerful brain-protective antioxidant.

Unfortunately, the bad oils create bad PR for all oils. Harmful oils, often used in processed foods, include soybean, corn, safflower, cottonseed, sunflower, palm, and any partially hydrogenated oils. All can increase LDL cholesterol and decrease HDL cholesterol. Canola oil, until recently recommended as a neutral choice, is implicated in increased Alzheimer's risk. If you see their names, run for your life!

FOR ADDED LIFE, PARTAKE OF
THESE TOP GOOD-GUY OILS:

1. MCT (medium-chain triglyceride) oil increases cognitive function, helps with weight management, supports gut health, and fights inflammation.

2. Omega-3 fish oil improves heart, brain, and skeletal health.

3. Olive oil improves cognitive function, cardiovascular function, and blood flow.

4. Hemp seed oil, with its perfect balance of omega fatty acids 3, 6, and 9, supports heart health and thicker, shinier hair, softer skin, and stronger nails.

5. Avocado oil offers nourishing antioxidants like vitamin E and is an awesome skin booster, which helps you age nicely on the outside, too.

6. Coconut oil gets mixed reviews as a healthy superfood, but it's universally loved as a terrific topical healing aid for common skin issues.

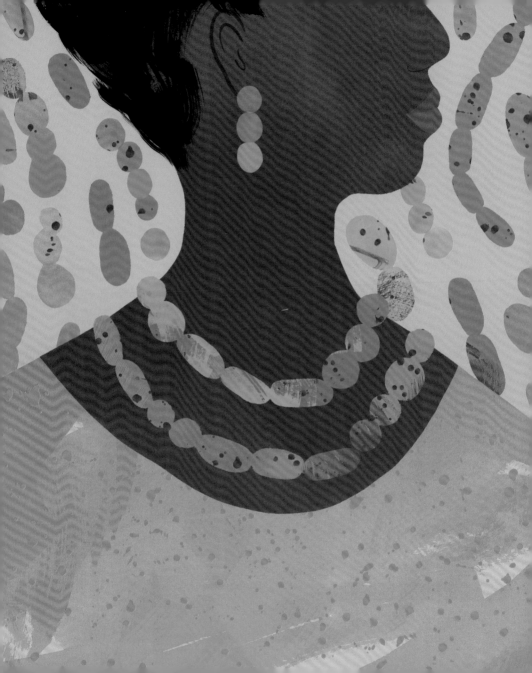

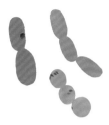

14

BE PRO-PROBIOTIC

Have you ever noticed that after a big meal your brain feels foggy? That's because of the interconnections between your gut and brain. In fact, poor gut health is now being linked to a variety of mental issues, including dementia, mood, and overall clarity.

On the flip side, good gut health is now being linked to improved mental health and a longer life, according to a study performed by the Buck Institute for Research on Aging.

Why? Quite simply, a badly functioning gut messes with your immune system, which in turn can cause a variety of major chronic degenerative diseases: diabetes, cancer, cardiovascular disease, and metabolic syndrome.

Basically, the better your gut health, the better your immune system, and thus the better your chances of a longer and

healthier life. So how do you achieve and maintain a healthy gut environment?

- Avoid inflammatory foods. These include sugar, fried foods, fast foods, processed foods, vegetable oils, artificial sweeteners, saturated fats, red meat, refined flours, and, for many of us, dairy.

- Eat lots of prebiotic and probiotic foods. Prebiotics behave like food for probiotics. Probiotics are beneficial bacteria that help keep your digestive system healthy by controlling growth of harmful bacteria.

RECOMMENDED PREBIOTICS: Asparagus, raw chicory root, raw Jerusalem artichoke, raw dandelion greens, raw garlic, raw leeks, raw or cooked onions, and raw jicama.

RECOMMENDED PROBIOTICS: Yogurt, kefir, sauerkraut, dark chocolate, miso soup, pickles, tempeh, and kombucha.

15

THE LONGER YOUR TELOMERES, THE LONGER YOUR LIFE

What the heck are telomeres?

Elizabeth Blackburn, a Nobel Prize–winning scientist, describes them this way: "If you think of your chromosomes—which carry your genetic material—as shoelaces, telomeres are the little protective tips at the end."

Blackburn warns that when your telomeres wear down and shorten, they stop being able to protect your chromosomes. As a result, your cells stop being able to replenish and wind up malfunctioning—thereby creating a wide variety of health issues, including cardiovascular disease, pulmonary fibrosis, depression, diabetes, vascular dementia, cancers, osteoporosis, and osteoarthritis.

So what's the short story on how to have long telomeres?

Blackburn says that you can lengthen your telomeres (or at least stop them from shortening) by

- Eating a diet plentiful in whole foods, omega-3 fatty acids, oily fish, and flaxseeds.
- Mindfully managing stress.

In fact, a variety of studies report that our telomere shortness is intrinsically related to how frequently and deeply we experiences stress.

A GOOD WAY TO REDUCE STRESS: Exercise! Studies report that if you put in a mere ten to fifteen minutes of light exercise a day you can help beef up your telomeres. Likewise, there's a strong correlation of shorter telomeres found in people who are very sedentary. So there should be no "buts" about getting off your butt!

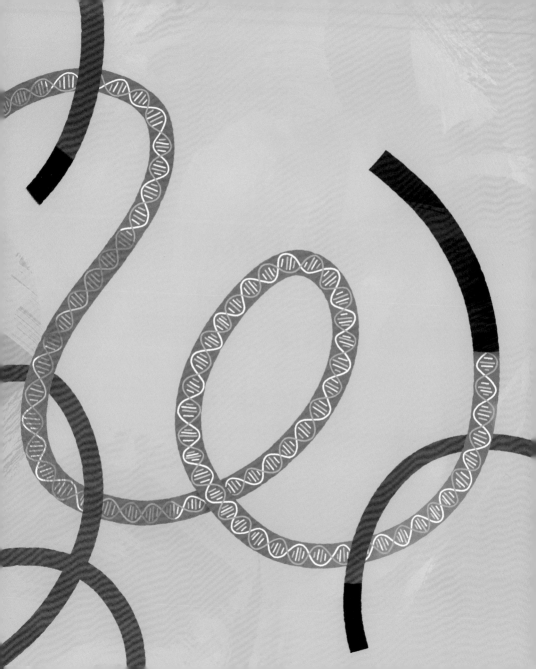

Eating
old food
will make
you older

16

EATING OLD FOOD WILL MAKE YOU OLDER

Question: What do you do when you notice a loaf of bread has been loafing around in your kitchen a little too long?

Do you still eat it—and just rip off any moldy edges?

If so, watch out! This older food could be making you older.

Studies show that eating food that's a li'l bit spoiled can actually age your cells and hurt your longevity.

The scoop: Researchers at Harvard Medical School performed a series of experiments on yeast, fruit flies, and mice. They discovered that if the flies and mice ate "older components," their lives were about 10 percent shorter than those who ate "fresher components."

Scientists believe the same holds true for us humans. If we make a habit of eating food on the older side, we speed the aging of our cells—and hurt our life expectancy.

LESSON LEARNED: If you don't want to expire sooner, pay attention to when your food is expiring! Even better, seek out super-fresh food sources like farmers' markets, home gardens, and local producers.

17

ADD SUPPLEMENTS
TO ADD YEARS TO YOUR LIFE

It's always better to get your vitamins from real-deal food than from a bottle. That said, here are three doctor-recommended supplements.

VITAMIN D_3

The *American Journal of Public Health* warns: "People with low blood levels of vitamin D_3 are more likely to die prematurely." According to a *Journal of Neurology* study, adults moderately deficient in vitamin D_3 had a 53 percent increased risk of getting dementia. Boosting vitamin D_3 has proven benefits: cancer patients with higher levels of vitamin D_3 tend to live longer and remain in remission longer than deficient patients (according to a study published in the *Journal of Clinical Endocrinology & Metabolism*). Make sure your D_3 includes K_2, which works like a traffic cop to ensure the right amounts of D_3 go to the right places in your body.

COQ_{10}

$CoQ_{10,}$ which stands for coenzyme Q_{10}, is a supplement that is well known for protecting your heart, lungs, brain, immune system—nearly every body cell. It basically helps your mitochondria burn fuel more effectively. Growing evidence shows CoQ_{10} can extend the life span of both primitive animals and mammals.

GREEN TEA EXTRACT

This gives your body a quick, easy boost of antioxidants, which reduce oxidative stress by fighting cell damage caused by pesky free radicals. And the catechins in green tea extract help reduce blood pressure, improve blood fat levels, boost heart health, enhance skin, power up memory—even help reduce cancer risk.

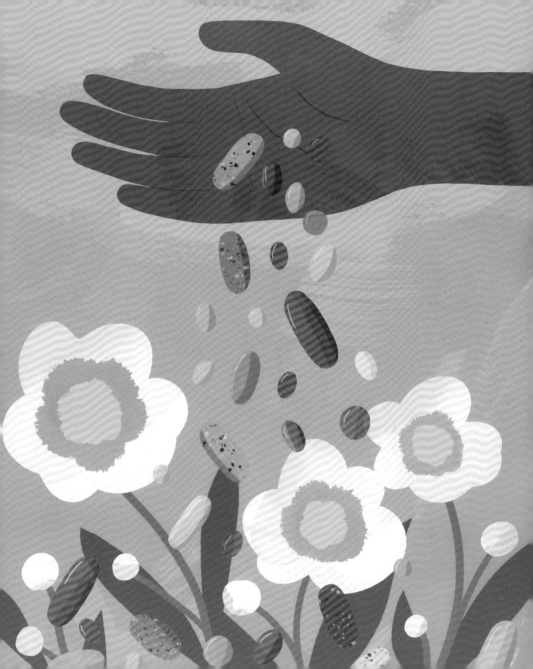

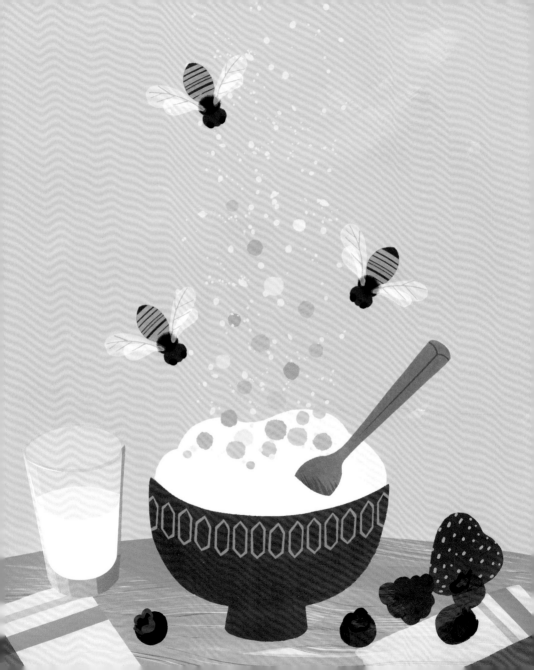

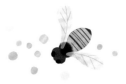

HEY, HONEY! TRY BEE POLLEN!

Bee pollen has been hailed by many nutritionists and scientists alike as a longevity superfood, prized for its multitudinous healing properties.

An amazing thing about bee pollen: it contains all of the nutrients you need to live.

Some studies have even shown that mice who were fed only bee pollen showed no signs of malnourishment.

BEE POLLEN CONSISTS OF:

- 55 percent carbohydrates
- 35 percent protein
- 3 percent vitamins and minerals
- 2 percent fatty acids
- 14.2 percent fiber
- Five to seven times the amino acids found in equal weights of beef, milk, eggs, or cheese
- High levels of vitamin B complex
- Any antioxidants, including lycopene, selenium, beta-carotene
- Vitamin C
- Vitamin E
- Lecithin—shown to normalize cholesterol and triglycerides

If you are interested in enjoying bee pollen, first make sure you're not allergic. Look for bee pollens with a large variety of colors (bright yellow, red, purple, green, brown, orange).

HOW TO ENJOY:

- Use as a topping over yogurt, cereal, even salads or popcorn!
- Blend ground pollen or granules into a smoothie.
- Incorporate into raw protein bars, raw desserts, or candies.

19

WINE GETS BETTER WITH AGE—
AND YOU AGE BETTER WITH WINE

If you want someone to toast you on your one-hundredth birthday, it might help if you start practicing toasting now!

According to the UC Irvine landmark 90+ Study, people who drink moderate amounts of alcohol are more likely to make it to age one hundred than folks who abstain.

A new study in the *Journal of the American College of Cardiology* offers this news: light to moderate alcohol use is associated with a reduced risk of death compared with no alcohol consumption at all. The study emphasizes that light alcohol consumption can reduce risk of death, while heavy consumption can have the opposite effect.

In particular, red wine is consistently reported to offer antiaging effects—credited to the antioxidant color pigment resveratrol found in the grape skins.

A study on mice at Harvard Medical School found that injecting the rodents with resveratrol increased their life span by a humongous 25 percent.

Resveratrol also has been reported to increase memory, reduce fat cells, inhibit cancer, and combat vascular disease and brain deterioration—according to neurosurgeon Joseph Maroon, whose book *The Longevity Factor* explains the link between wine and a longer life.

If you're not a lover of red wine, no worries! The antiaging benefits of resveratrol are also found in peanut butter, dark chocolate, blueberries, and (of course) red grapes!

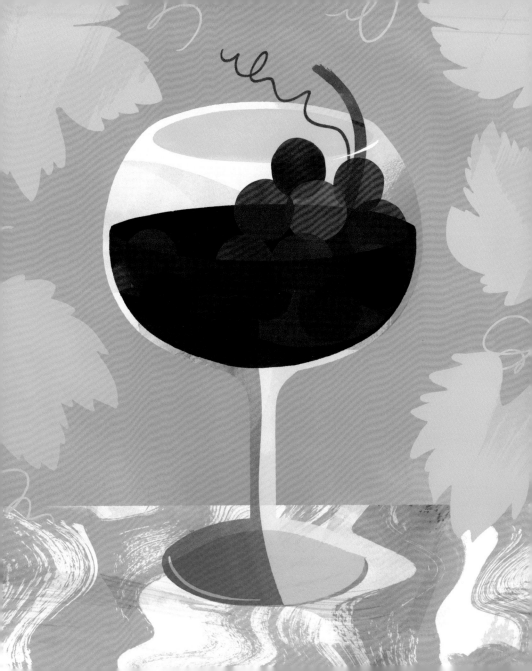

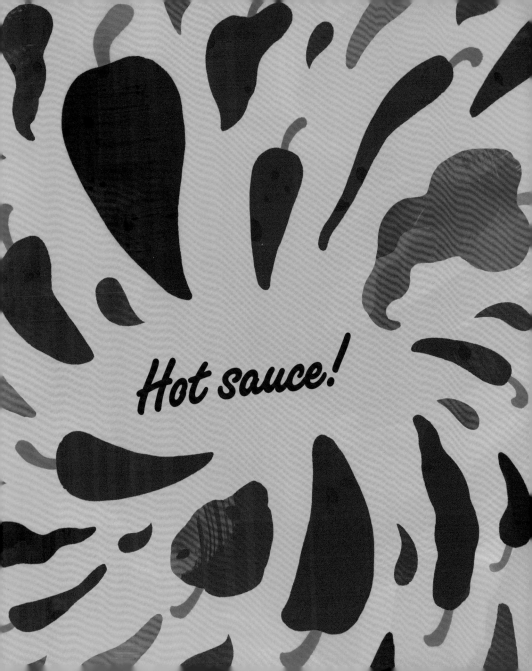

Hot sauce!

20

A SECRET SAUCE FOR A LONGER LIFE: HOT SAUCE!

This unusual chili pepper–touting longevity advice is backed up by research.

University of California professor Andrew Dillin studied mice who were bred without a specific pain sensor called TRPV1. These lucky mice wound up living longer and were less likely to develop age-related diseases.

David Sinclair of Harvard Medical School was impressed by Dillin's findings, saying, "It is striking that the mice without TRPV1 were protected from some of the ravages of old age, including declines in metabolism, cognition, and physical activity."

As it turns out, there's a molecule found in chili peppers, called capsaicin, that can mimic the same benefits of losing this TRPV1 pain receptor.

Meaning? When you regularly indulge in chilli peppers, you're getting lots of this capsaicin—so you get the same positive longevity perks as losing TRPV1.

In summary: all this good longevity news makes hot peppers extra hot stuff!

SO HOW MUCH EXTRA SPICINESS DO YOU NEED? According to Lu Qi, an associate professor at the Harvard School of Public Health who recently published a study on this topic in the *BMJ*, try eating one to five more spicy meals each week.

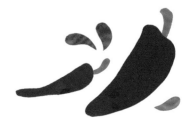

21

GET HOOKED ON FISH

A Harvard School of Public Health study showed that older people with the highest levels of omega-3s have life spans longer by 2.2 years (on average) than those with low omega-3 blood levels.

Sound fishy to you? Well, it's true!

Why? Heart attacks and strokes are the world's leading causes of death. And omega-3 fatty acids have been shown to have numerous benefits for heart health by helping improve levels of triglycerides, blood pressure, HDL cholesterol, blood clots, plaque, and inflammation.

So, how do you go about getting your omega-3s? Get more fishy! Give a starring role on your plate to oily and fatty fish.

FISH HIGH IN OMEGA-3S:

- wild-caught Alaskan salmon
- Pacific Coast salmon
- herring
- lake trout
- sardines

HEADS UP! If you're going to indulge in tuna, keep away from canned white tuna, which is albacore. It has mercury levels almost three times higher than the smaller skipjack tuna used for most canned light tuna—the far safer choice. The following fish species are reported to be high in mercury, so you should avoid them: king mackerel, marlin, orange roughy, shark, swordfish, tilefish, ahi tuna, and bigeye tuna.

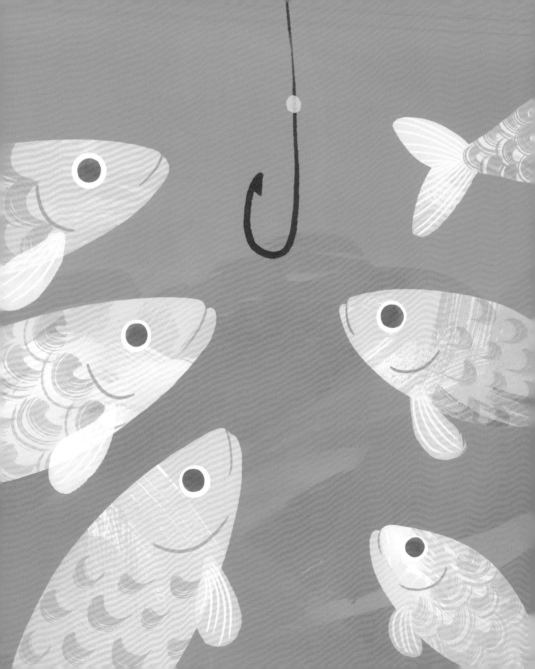

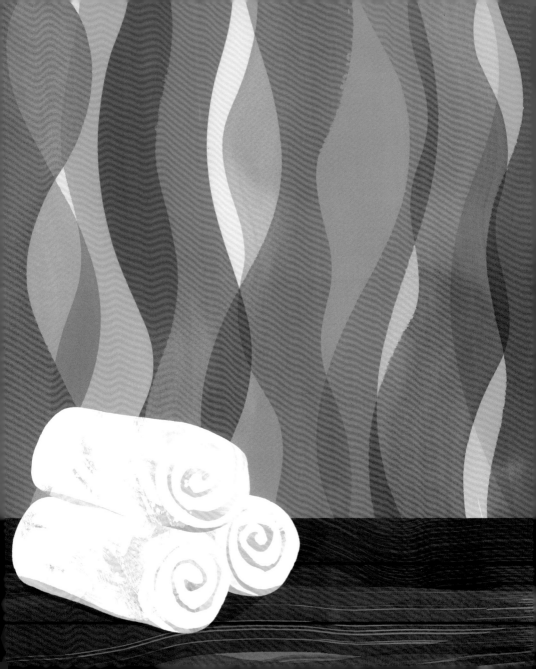

22

TURN UP THE HEAT

Here's a fun longevity tip, which is actually a bit on the lazy side: Go hang out in a sauna!

According to a study in the journal *JAMA Internal Medicine*, you can reduce your risk of a number of cardiovascular conditions (including heart failure and coronary heart disease) simply by shvitzing it up in a sauna.

How can this be?

Saunas mimic the results of light or moderate exercise—increasing heart rate and boosting sweatiness.

Plus, saunas help relax you—and stress reduction is always a helpful life span increaser.

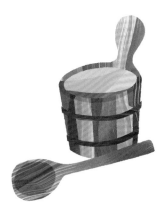

23

DANCE YOUR WAY TO
A LONGER LIFE

Want to know some good steps to a longer life? Try some tango, hip hop, or salsa steps!

Yep, there's a wide range of dancing steps to get your groove on—and a wide range of reasons why you should try them!

- Regular dancing can help reduce your risk of cardiovascular disease, high blood pressure, type 2 diabetes, and perhaps some cancers. Says who? Dr. Peter Mace, assistant medical director of Bupa Wellness.

- Dancing alleviates social isolation. Research by Dr. Jonathan Skinner of Queen's University Belfast says the social benefits of dancing help counteract aging.

- Dancing gives you an energizing "dancer's high," which can satisfy the craving for less healthy habits. Researchers from Budapest and from Trent University in Nottingham, UK, developed a standardized tool called the Dance Motivation Inventory, or DMI. These researchers found that people who dance do it to gain mood enhancement, escape stress, and increase socialization—the same rewards people seek when pursuing riskier behaviors like drinking and gambling.

- Dancing is one of the most effective physical activities out there to slow down the aging process of the brain. According to a study in *Frontiers in Human Neuroscience*, this is because it requires memorizing new steps, movements, and routines.

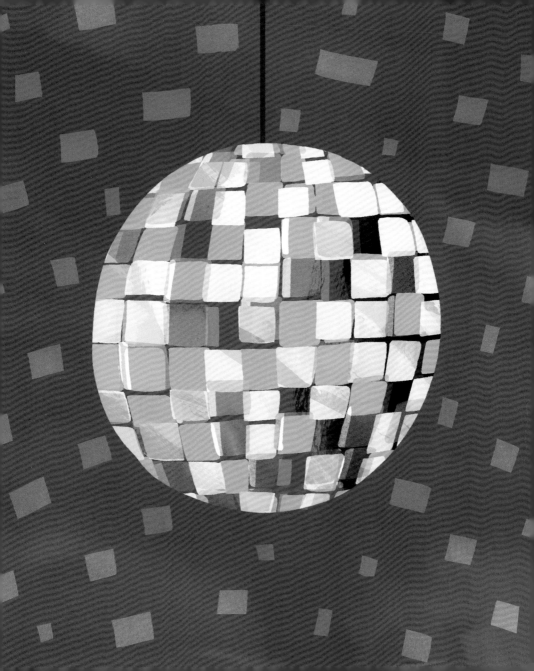

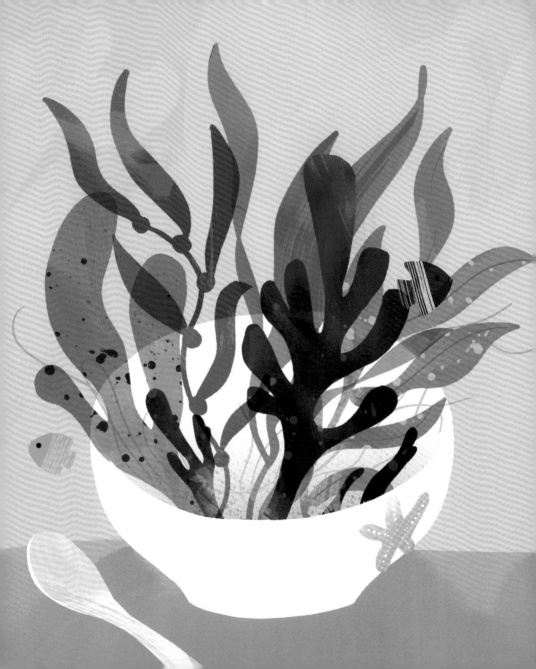

24

KELP CAN HELP

Your health is affected not only by what you eat but also by what you do *not* eat.

If you're presently *not* regularly chowing down on seaweed, marine algae, and sea vegetables, then you're missing out on an ocean of health boosters.

In fact, researchers on the Blue Zone Japanese island of Okinawa credit the inhabitants' habit of eating sea vegetables as one reason for their longevity.

There's real science behind the longevity perks of eating sea veggies. They're loaded with trace minerals that are super essential to health. In fact, research shows the body cannot dispose of acid unless it has minerals to aid the process. Basically, acid needs a "mineral chaperone." Without minerals, the body's acid-alkaline balance can skew to the acid side, as acidity becomes entrenched. Dr. Gary Price Todd, a physician and expert on degenerative and age-related diseases, says, "The lack of minerals is the root of all disease."

SOME RECOMMENDED SEA VEGGIES TO EXPLORE:

- wakame
- hijiki
- arame
- dulse
- kelp
- kombu
- spirulina

BONUS: Sea vegetables are not only high in minerals and trace minerals—they're also loaded with beneficial enzymes, coenzymes, vitamins, chlorophyll, growth hormones, and phytonutrients.

25

WASH YOUR HANDS

This longevity tip wins hands down: Make sure you put your hands down in a sink before eating!

This familiar mom-knows-best recommendation is not only easy and simple to do but could actually save your life!

In fact, according to the World Health Organization, making a habit of regular handwashing could save more lives around the world than any vaccine or other medical intervention. The Centers for Disease Control and Prevention (CDC) also urges people to wash their hands—concurring that this simple act is one of the most effective things we can do to prevent the spread of infectious diseases.

A study from Michigan State University reported that, shockingly, 95 percent of people right here in the United States do not wash their hands properly. The researchers sneakily observed 3,749 people in various post-flush restroom scenarios. They discovered that 95 percent showed a "widespread disregard" for bathroom washing etiquette. Twenty-three percent washed without soap. (Eccchh.) Ten percent didn't wash their hands at all. (Yikes!)

WHAT TO DO? Proper handwashing means that you use both soap and water and wash for at least thirty seconds. An easy timer trick: Sing "Happy Birthday" twice through—then get ready to celebrate more birthdays, knowing that you're protecting yourself against dangerous bacteria!

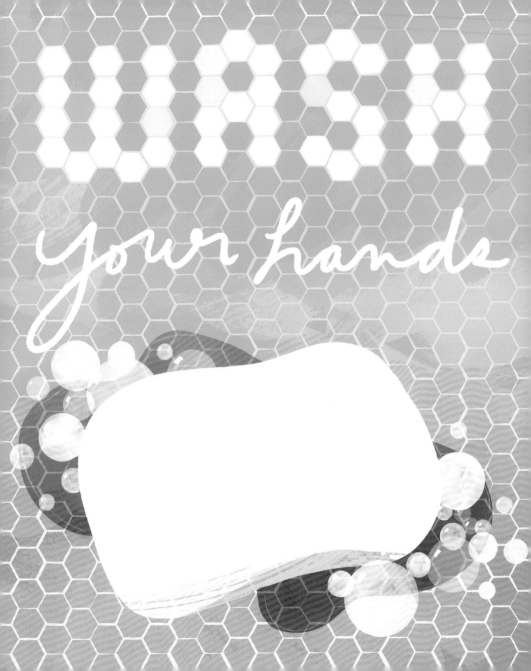

WASH

your hands

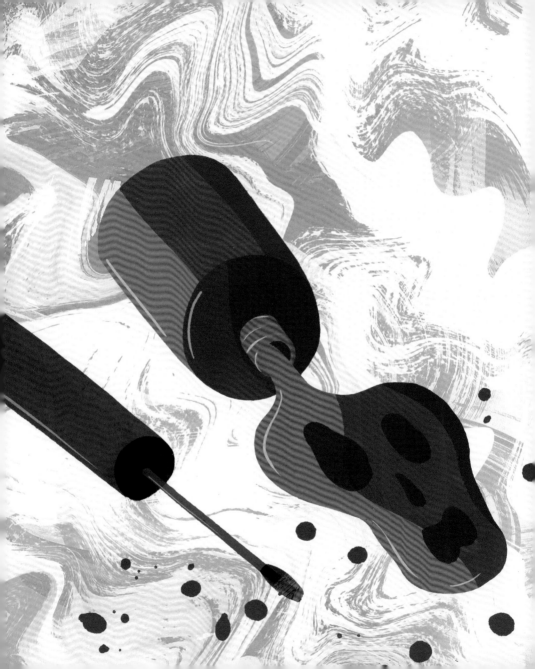

26

STOP DYEING TO BE BEAUTIFUL

You know those beautifully colored polishes women love to paint on their fingers and tootsies? Many are lady killers.

Dr. Thu Quach, of Stanford University and the Cancer Prevention Institute of California, says the chemicals in many polishes lead to many issues: cancer, infertility, hormonal disruption, thinking and memory problems, nausea, respiratory problems, uncontrollable muscle contractions, headaches, and then some.

Researchers at Duke University are also alarmed by how quickly the dangerous chemicals found in polishes are absorbed into the body. They found that women who use nail polish wound up having a dangerous chemical in their bodies called TPHP—just ten to fourteen hours after painting their nails.

Unfortunately, there are a range of bad-guy chemicals to look out for in a range of beauty products—in everything from hair dye to makeup to perfume to deodorant.

BEFORE YOU BUY ANY BEAUTY PRODUCTS, WATCH OUT FOR THESE BEASTLY INGREDIENTS:

- Formaldehyde—carcinogen
- Toluene—additive in gasoline
- Phthalates—endocrine disruptor
- Polyethylene glycol (PEG)—skin carcinogen
- Phenoxyethanol—nervous system depressant
- Fragrance—linked to cancer, birth defects, and central nervous system disorders
- Avobenzone—causes cell mutation
- PABA and PABA esters—cause damage to DNA

27

WHAT YOU DON'T SEE
CAN KILL YOU

You know that scary shower scene in the classic movie *Psycho*? It turns out the Janet Leigh character had more to worry about than her attacker. Her vinyl shower curtain was a threat too!

Studies including one by the Center for Health, Environment & Justice report how the chemicals used in vinyl shower curtains can cause serious damage to the liver and the nervous, reproductive, and respiratory systems.

Why? When heated, vinyl shower curtains release dangerous chemicals into the air. The solution? Trade in your cheap vinyl curtain for a cloth one—or invest in a glass shower door. (Bonus: Get an air purifier to catch those nasties—and avoid becoming the one out of eight annual global deaths due to air pollution, according to the World Health Organization!)

ALAS, MORE INVISIBLE TOXIN DANGERS LURK IN SEEMINGLY INNOCENT PLACES:

- Plastic-bottled water. Chemicals in the plastic can leach into the water and cause a variety of health issues.

- The sun's UV rays. These are linked to skin cancer and a range of eye issues. The solar solution? Invest in wraparound sunglasses and a good sunscreen with zinc and titanium minerals, not dangerous oxybenzone and/or retinyl palmitate.

- X-rays. The WHO and the U.S. government consider X-rays a carcinogen, proven to cause DNA mutations leading to cancer later in life. Talk to your doctor about limiting your exposure.

- Loud music. Preserve your long-term hearing; don't crank up the volume of your favorite music. Some studies link hearing loss with the risk of dementia or Alzheimer's, says otolaryngologist Dr. Frank R. Lin of the National Institute on Aging. The Hearing, Health and Technology Matters organization reports a link between healthy hearing and healthy living, noting that hearing loss can lead to depression, cognitive decline, and social isolation.

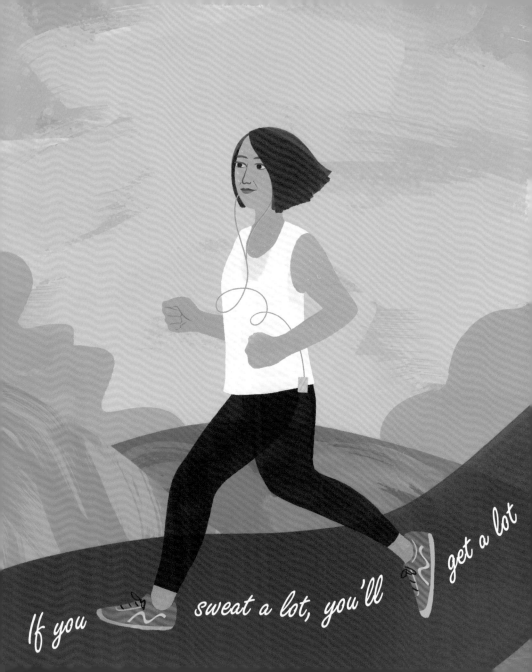

If you sweat a lot, you'll get a lot

28

IF YOU SWEAT A LOT, YOU'LL GET A LOT

Think you don't have time to work out?

Well, working out will automatically give you more time—around four to five years more time tagged onto your life! And that's a consistently researched fact.

The National Cancer Institute reported that simply meeting the World Health Organization's recommendation of 150 minutes of exercise a week can add up to 4.5 years to your life, compared to never exercising.

Meaning? The time spent working out has a very good Return on Investment!

A good trick to working out more? "Pick fun workouts—with terrific music—workouts which challenge you to push yourself further," recommends Fred DeVito, cofounder and EVP of Exhale Spa.

Fred also reports that the sweatier and stinkier the workout, the greater the benefits for longevity.

"The goal is to get your heart rate up to a place where you feel a little breathless, but you're still able to talk," explains Fred. "Basically, when you raise your heart rate, you're exercising your heart, building new blood vessels and mitochondria, increasing your oxygen-carrying blood flow capacity, burning fat, and building muscle."

These are a few of my favorite things!

Need a little extra kick in the tush to get to the gym?

READ THIS SENTENCE OVER AND OVER: The American Heart Association says that being physically active is a key factor in preventing the nation's #1 and #5 killers—heart disease and stroke!

29

GARLIC: BAD FOR VAMPIRES, GOOD FOR HUMANS

Garlic might be detrimental to the life of vampires, but as long as you're human, garlic can help you live longer and healthier.

Garlic's been considered a super food since super long ago. In ancient Greece and Rome, folks thought garlic boosted strength and endurance. Olympic Greek athletes even used to chow down on garlic before their big games to empower their performance. And builders of the Egyptian pyramids used to gobble garlic to increase their lifting abilities.

So, what did those ancient folks intuitively know—which modern scientists can now back up with facts?

According to research at the University of Alabama at Birmingham, garlic does boost energy and health, thanks to the hydrogen sulfide gas it creates. When released into your body, hydrogen sulfide relaxes blood vessels, which in turn allows more oxygen to travel to your organs.

The perks: Garlic lowers high blood pressure and protects the body against cardiovascular disease.

Many Chinese researchers love garlic's hydrogen sulfide for the body so much that they've called it "the key to a longer life."

WHAT TO DO? The most potent kind of garlic to eat is from bulbs that have begun to sprout. After you cut, crush, or mince it, let it sit for five to ten minutes, so as to release its healthy compounds. Oh, and don't get lazy and rely on garlic powder, which does *not* contain allicin— the source of garlic's key health benefits.

INTERESTING SIDE NOTE: The reason garlic is good for you is also the reason it gives you bad breath. Hydrogen sulfide gives off a strong sulfur odor. The solution? Studies have found that eating an apple or lettuce after eating garlic helps improve your breath.

flower

stalk

bulb

clove

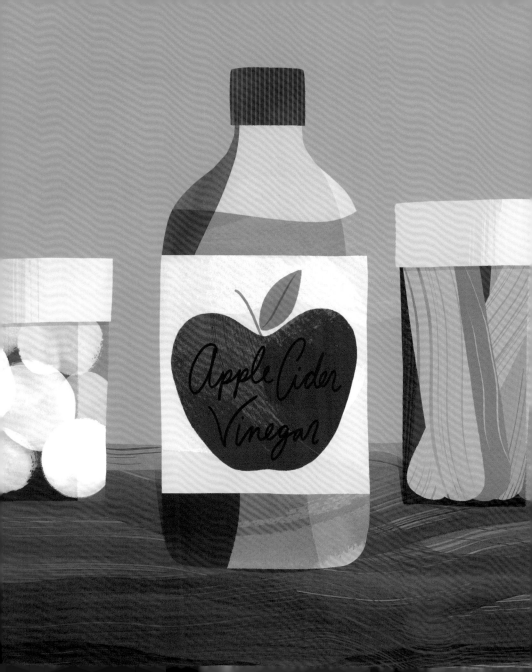

30

AN APPLE CIDER VINEGAR A DAY KEEPS THE DOCTOR AWAY

Nutritionist Danielle Pashko recommends starting the day with a tall glass of water with about one tablespoon of apple cider vinegar.

This admittedly tangy drink offers many good life boosters. In 2016, a study by Michael Mosley and Aston University showed that drinking diluted apple cider vinegar appeared to lower blood sugar levels.

The American Diabetes Association reports that taking two tablespoons of apple cider vinegar before bed can reduce fasting blood sugars—and that having less than an ounce of apple cider vinegar with a high-carb meal helps control insulin.

Plus, research has found that the acetic acid found in apple cider vinegar lowers cholesterol and triglyceride levels, reduces blood pressure, helps control appetite, and aids digestion and absorption of minerals like calcium (which helps you get more health benefits out of your food).

BIG REMINDER: Always dilute apple cider vinegar by adding only one tablespoon to a tall glass of water. If you don't dilute it enough, it can cause stomach issues and tooth enamel erosion.

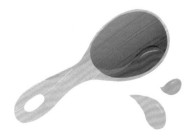

31

AVOID THIS STRIP ACT

All white rice begins as brown rice. However, once its outer coating of bran is hulled off, white rice becomes stripped of its beneficial nutrients, fiber, vitamins, minerals, potassium, magnesium, phosphorus, lignans, and phytoestrogens—basically all its goodies.

Trust me: this is a strip act you don't want to have any part of.

If you want to live a long life, keep your rice brown—and cash in on the following longevity perks:

- Brown rice contains more than seventy antioxidants, including beloved age-defying fighters like vitamin E and CoQ_{10}.

- One cup of brown rice gives you 88 percent of your daily value for manganese, which boosts perky sex hormones and helps with cholesterol.

- Brown rice is high in selenium, which has been shown to induce DNA repair—believed to help with cancer prevention.

- Brown rice helps lower your type 2 diabetes risk. Why? Unlike white rice, brown rice is very fibrous, so it gets digested slowly and your sugar level doesn't rise so speedily.

- A cup of brown rice provides 14 percent of your daily value for fiber, which helps protect against colon cancer, high cholesterol, and atherosclerosis.

Be sure to choose whole-grain options in a whole lot of other foods—like breads, pastas, and cereals. The same perks of reduced illness and increased longevity apply. As *Forbes* health investigator Alice G. Walton reminds us: "The chunkier and wilder the grains, the better."

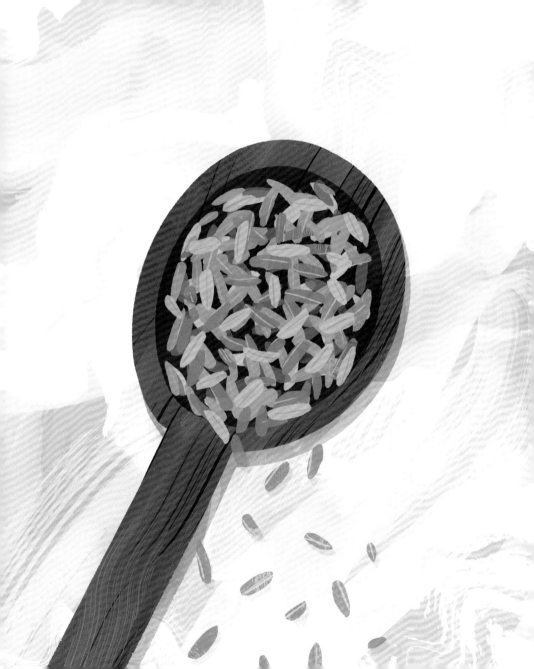

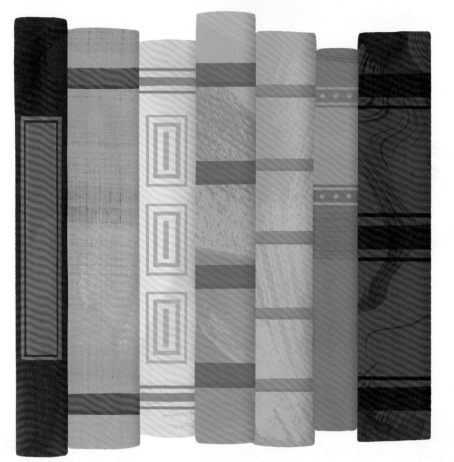

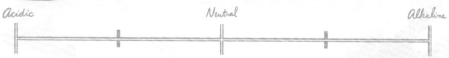

Acidic   Neutral   Alkaline

GET A PHD IN YOUR PH LEVELS

Acid rain is bad for the environment. And acidic foods are bad for your body's environment.

When your body has an acidic pH level below 7.0, it means you're increasing your body's internal inflammation, which leads to a lowered immune function and greater risk of heart disease, cancer, and Alzheimer's.

An alkaline diet may result in a number of health benefits: improved bone health, reduced muscle wasting, boosted brain health, and less chance of chronic diseases such as hypertension and stroke.

The goal: Ideally, a slightly alkaline pH level of 7.4—or higher.

The plan? Try to eat an anti-inflammatory diet of 80 percent alkaline foods and 20 percent acidic foods, by following these recommendations:

- Don't eat—or try to limit—meat, sugar, dairy, white flour, white rice, animal fats, trans fats, processed and refined foods, commercial condiments, alcohol, ice cream, pizza, and canned foods.

- Load up on healthy fats, fish, nuts, seeds, legumes, leafy greens and salads, high-water foods, and fresh low-sugar fruits—preferably organically grown.

- Drink plenty of water each day— ideally half of your body weight (in pounds) in ounces. Feel free to squeeze a little lemon into your water. Lemon's actually alkalinizing!

I'm a coffee lover, so I was saddened to hear that coffee is acidic. Happily, there's the universal principle of "everything in moderation." So if you gotta drink your coffee, increase your alkaline levels elsewhere.

EXHALE STRESS, INHALE LONG LIFE

If you want to increase the amount of time you're breathing, you might want to take more time to breathe—specifically, in meditation.

According to researchers at Purdue University, worrying and feeling anxious can load you up with stress hormones, which leads to health issues like cardiovascular disease, gastrointestinal issues, weight problems, and even some cancers.

Happily, meditation can help reduce your stress and thereby breathe new life back into your life span!

Meditation has also been shown to slow aging by super-powering your brain. Researchers at the University of California and Harvard Medical School have compared the brains of meditators and nonmeditators and discovered that meditation could help slow structural degeneration of the brain's gray matter and white matter.

Translation: Meditation is good for your brain's cells, dendrites, axons, and synapses—all of which is good news for both your mind and your body.

HOW TO GET STARTED:

1. Decide how long you want to meditate. Set an alarm.

2. Find a cozy, quiet place. Sit comfortably.

3. Close your eyes and become aware of your breath. Breathe naturally for ten to twenty seconds.

4. After you become fully focused on your breathing, make an addition: when you exhale, think the words "Exhale stress," and when you inhale, think, "Inhale peace." Repeat until your timer sounds.

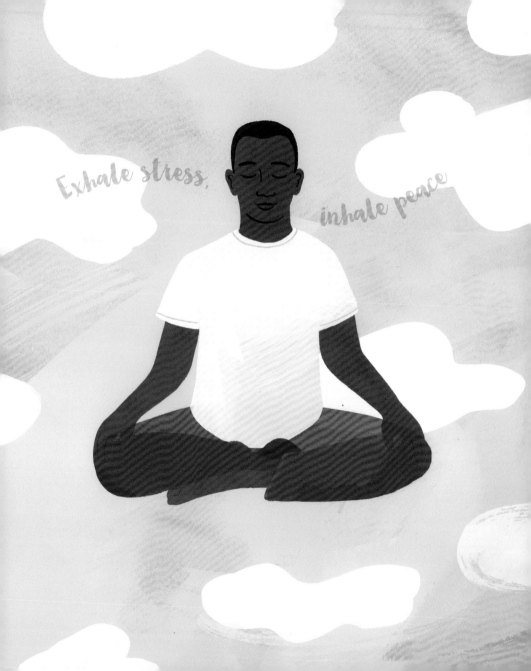

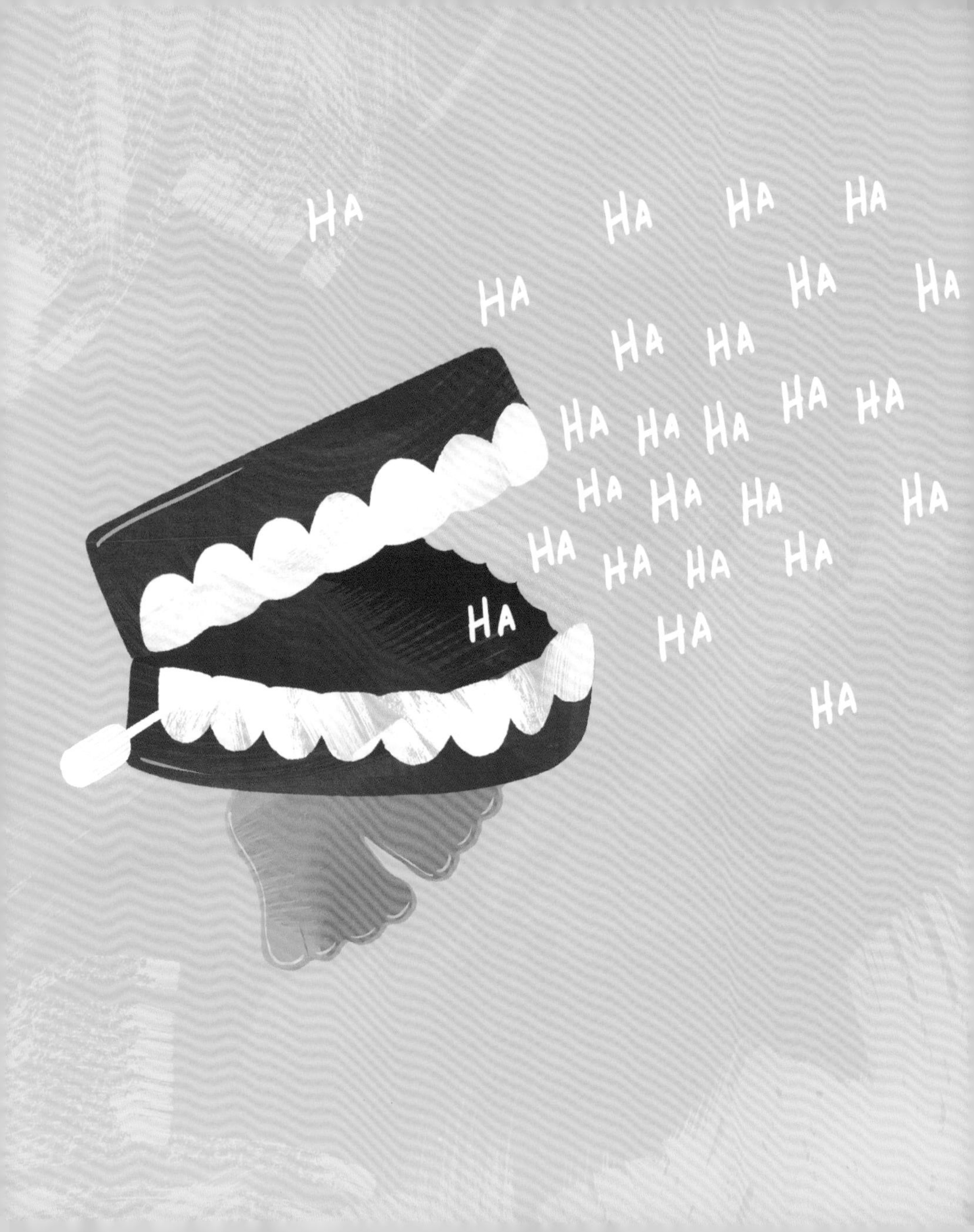
HA HA HA HA
HA HA HA
HA HA
HA HA HA HA HA
HA HA HA HA
HA HA HA HA
HA
HA
HA

TRY THE CHUCKLE PRESCRIPTION

Don't laugh, but research shows that laughter helps you live longer.

In particular, laughter has been shown to boost the immune system, increase natural killer cell activity in the blood, increase free radical–scavenging capacity in saliva, lower levels of the stress hormone cortisol, and control and reduce pain levels.

Another perk to giggling: A study from the Foundation for the Advancement of International Science (in Japan) showed that laughter seems to lower levels of a dangerous protein involved in the progression of diabetic nephropathy— the leading cause of kidney failure.

Another amazing laughter perk: Laughing can reduce inflammation— the culprit in a wide range of diseases, from arthritis to cancer. As a result, laughter can help reduce age-related chronic diseases, which are frequently caused by inflammation.

Funny but true story about laughter: Study results published in *Rheumatology* showed a significant drop in blood levels of key inflammatory compounds after rheumatoid arthritis patients watched a funny movie.

Scientific proof that laughter's good medicine: Researchers at Indiana State University recorded amounts of what they call "mirthful laughter" and found that levels of interleukin 6, a cytokine that plays a central role in inflammation, dropped significantly in arthritis patients, but not in a comparison group. The anti-inflammatory effects have also been shown to last for twelve hours after the laughter has subsided.

YOUR ASSIGNMENT: Do things that make you LOL!

THINKING OUTSIDE OF THE BOX CAN KEEP YOU OUTSIDE OF THAT OTHER BOX!

Do you show openness to novel ideas, creativity, or flexible thinking?

If so, you have an enhanced chance of living longer—according to research by Professor Nicholas Turiano, reported in the *Journal of Aging and Health*.

Openness and creativity show up in a range of studies (collected between 1990 and 2008) as key personality traits of people who not only lived longer but also showed lower metabolic risk and superior stress responses.

Why? "Creativity is protective of health because it draws on a variety of neural networks within the brain," explains Professor Turiano. "As a result, individuals high in creativity maintain the integrity of their neural networks—even into old age."

Basically, the brain is the command center for the rest of your body's functions. The more you exercise all parts of your brain, the better you help all parts of your body operate at their best.

Professor Turiano also believes creative people handle stress better because they're more likely to view problems as challenges or games to solve—and to want to problem-solve solutions rather than dwell on issues.

Openness is also expressed as a love for trying new things and being open to new beliefs and insights. Deepak Chopra said it well: "People don't grow old; when they stop growing, they become old."

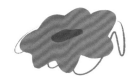

YOUR ASSIGNMENT:

Not naturally open-minded or creative? Fake the neural activity till you make the neural activity! Starting today, force yourself to regularly:

- Try new restaurants.

- Read editorials that go against your thinking.

- Pick up a new hobby.

- Do puzzle books and word association games.

- Draw in sketchbooks and coloring books—don't be afraid to color outside of the lines and make daring color choices!

- Be sure to ask these six questions a lot: Why? Where? When? Who? What? How?

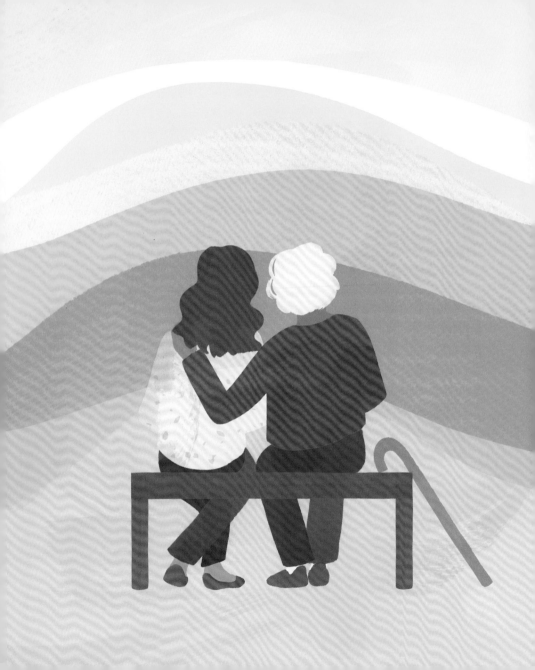

36

HELPING OTHERS HELPS YOU LIVE LONGER

Being blessed with a good strong aorta and nicely flowing arteries helps ensure that you'll live longer.

But guess what?

So does having a good *metaphorical* heart!

If you love helping others, you can help yourself to a bunch more extra years on this planet.

In fact, more than thirty study reports compiled by the Corporation for National and Community Service found that volunteering increases your life expectancy *significantly*. (Their word!)

Plus, a University of Michigan study backed up these thirty studies—supporting consistent findings that people who volunteer live longer than those who don't.

THERE'S ONE CATCH: The volunteering has to be done for the purpose of helping others—not just to help yourself!

37

BLESS YOUR STRESS

A small shift in your view of stress could make a huge difference in your lifeline.

In 2012, researchers from the University of Wisconsin-Madison performed a fascinating study on stress with about 28,000 people. The study found that having a combo of a lot of stress *and* also having a belief system that stress was hurting your health increased the risk of premature death by 43 percent.

Harvard researchers did a similar study—on three different groups of people. Each group was asked to talk in front of a bunch of grumpy evaluators. Afterward, they were given a complicated word test.

Before this secret stress test, the first group was told to play fun video games. The second group was told to pay no attention to their anxiety. And the third group was given some unusual info about the benefits of stress: that stress symptoms

(higher heart rate, faster breathing, and internal jitters) are all biological benefits for making you stronger, faster, smarter, better! In essence, stress evolved to help us get through such events—and come out on top.

This third group, having learned to "bless their stress," were more successful at their speeches and were rated as more confident. Plus, physiologically, they wound up managing their stress response far better than the other groups.

YOUR ASSIGNMENT:

- Stop thinking: *"Stress is increasing my risk for cardiovascular disease and heart attack."*

- Start thinking: *"Stress is helping my heart work harder, and it's speeding up my breathing so more oxygen gets to my brain so I can think more clearly."*

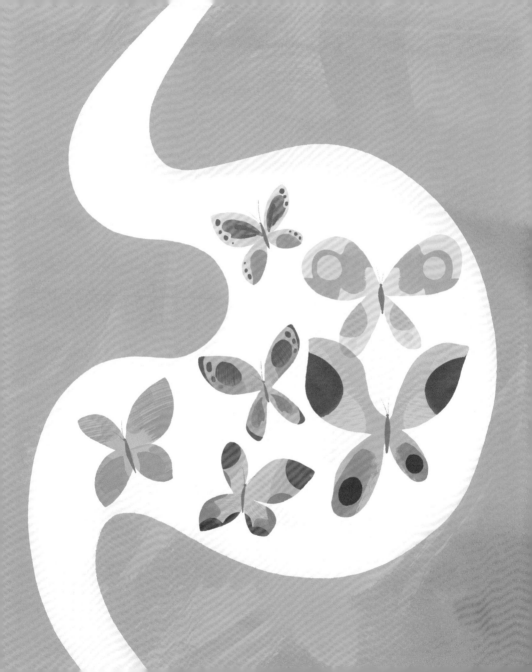

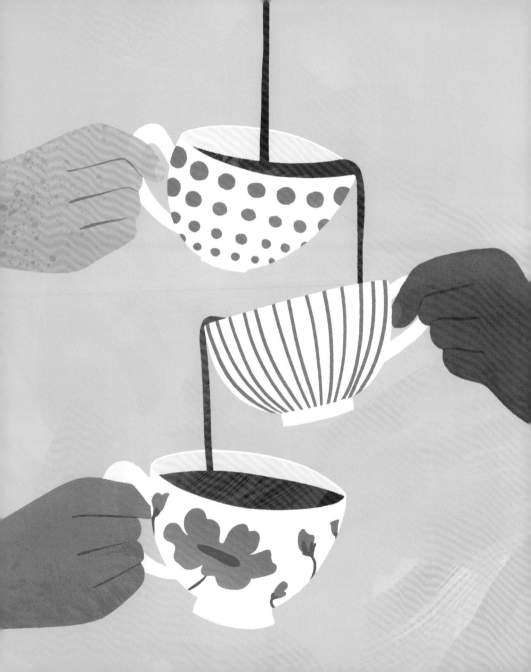

THE BETTER YOUR SOCIAL LIFE, THE LONGER YOUR WHOLE LIFE!

If you want to live longer, friend up!

In 2010, researchers at Brigham Young University published a fascinating study: People who enjoyed strong social ties had a 50 percent increased likelihood of survival over a period of 7.5 years in comparison to folks with weak or no social ties.

In the journal *PLoS Medicine*, BYU professors report the many longevity risks of "low social interaction." They went so far as to compare the "low level socializing" to these well-known risk factors and found them:

- Equivalent to smoking fifteen cigarettes a day.
- More harmful than not exercising.

Lynne C. Giles, a longevity researcher from Flinders University, reports that close family ties don't affect longevity in the same powerful ways that friendships do. "By differentiating between friends, children and other relatives," Giles says, "we were able to show that it is friends, rather than children or relatives, which confer the most benefit to survival later in life."

WARNING: Too *many* friends could be bad for your health and mood. According to Robin Dunbar, an Oxford University researcher, in order to cash in on the goodies of friendship, you should focus on five good friends—and cap your tribe at a maximum of 150.

YOUR ASSIGNMENT: If you want the health perks of friendship, be sure to focus on quality—not quantity—connections.

ONE OF THE BEST DOCTORS HAS FOUR LEGS

Dogs and cats are easy to love. Now here's another reason to love having an adorable pet around your home.

Research shows that both cat and dog owners tend to be healthier and live longer than their petless peers.

The *Medical Journal of Australia* reported that pet owners generally have lower blood pressure and triglyceride and cholesterol levels than petless peeps.

The American Heart Association reports that owning a dog lowers your risk of cardiovascular disease and speeds recovery from heart attacks. And a Minnesota Stroke Institute study reported that owning a cat significantly decreases your chance of dying from heart disease.

A Rutgers University study reported that pet owners have significantly fewer sick days per year than non-pet owners.

Dr. Andrea Beetz and colleagues at Rostock University discovered that owning a pet reduces cortisol in your body, thereby helping your immune functions.

Good news! You don't have to own a pet to boost your health.

Wilkes University reported that students who simply petted a dog for eighteen minutes had elevated immunoglobulins (aka antibodies).

YOUR ASSIGNMENT: If you want to live a furry long time, hang out with a furry friend.

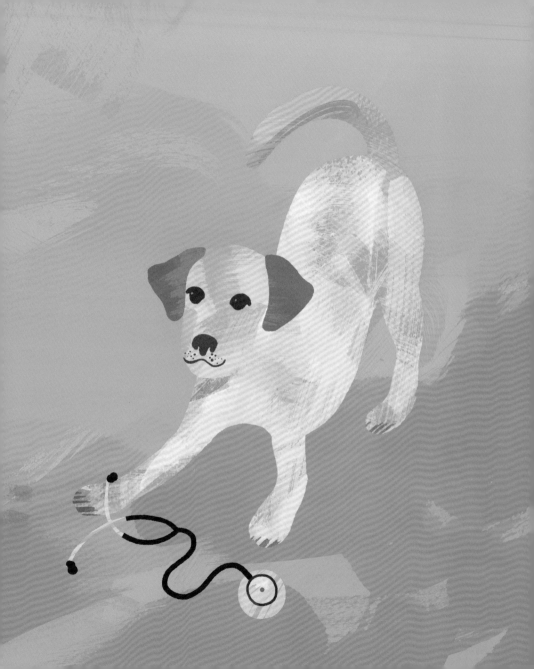

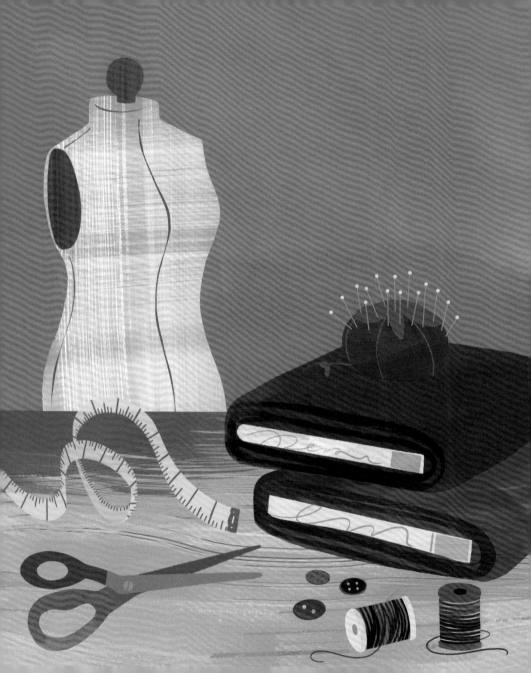

40

DELAY WHEN YOU RETIRE, DELAY WHEN YOU EXPIRE

If you want to keep on living, you might want to keep on making a living.

According to Harvard's famed Longevity Project, those who made it further into old age were folks who enjoyed fulfilling careers and continued to work—at least part time—well into their seventies.

Plus, if you read my intro, you'll remember that *plan de vida* (translated as "reason to live") is a common philosophy of spritely elders living in Nicoya, Costa Rica—a famed centenarian hot spot. These centenarians credit their longevity to "living with a purpose."

Peter Flax interviewed a range of incredible older showbiz folks for the *Hollywood Reporter*, many of whom were still actively working well into their nineties—or further. These celebs agreed that their passionate work "kept them in good spirits and out of assisted living."

- The brilliant Stan Lee (ninety-three at the time) said: "If anybody forced me to play golf for a few hours a day, I'd shoot 'em. What could be more fun than coming up with stories?"

- The always cheery Betty White (ninety-four at the time) said: "When you're doing something you love to do, that's got to be a healthy thing."

- Genius writer Carl Reiner (then ninety-five) called the idea of retiring "a joke." He says he's "too busy to die"—and even wrote a book with that as the title!

41

MINDFULLY CREATE YOUR FOOD COMMANDMENTS

Quick Quiz:

Do you tend to stop eating when . . .

- you're feeling full—because you're eating mindfully.
- your plate is empty—because you're not paying attention to your thoughts or body signals?

If the latter, your health is at risk—because when you zone out, you make stupider health choices.

Brian Wansink, PhD, has conducted studies at Cornell University showing how and why people wind up overstuffing themselves. He's famous for fooling subjects into consuming multiple quarts of soup—because he fed them from trick bottomless bowls. They kept mindlessly spooning up their soup without ever realizing their tummies were full.

The cure for mindless eating?

Dr. Wansink suggests creating an ongoing food policy, or what I like to refer to as my personal "food commandments": a list of intentions I remember before every meal—and stick to. Feel free to use them as thy own!

- Thou shalt put down thy fork every minute or so while eating—and take full pleasure in thy food.
- Thou shalt take time to do a quick check-in with thy body ten minutes into a meal.
- Thou shalt eat only raw veggies and hummus in front of thy TV—and never chips.
- Thou shalt be the first person to order at a restaurant—to avoid the temptation to copy others' unhealthy food choices.

- Thou shalt never eat pretzels directly from the bag or ice cream directly from the pint. Instead, thou shalt put portion-controlled quantities directly into a bowl.

- Thou shalt identify thy emotional state when feeling hungry—and make sure it is not sadness or stress that is inspiring eating a bowl of chips.

- Thou shalt drink a glass of water when feeling hungry—and make sure it is not merely dehydration that is inspiring eating a bowl of pretzels.

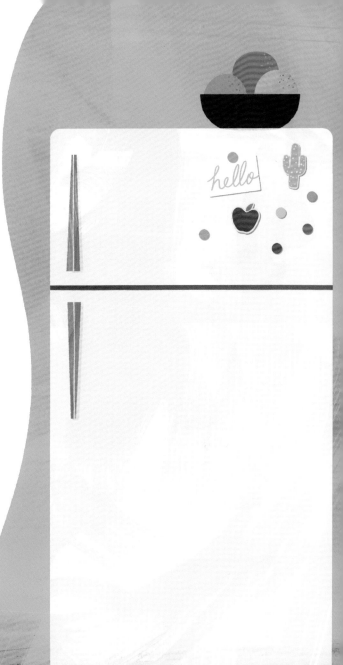

Lie about your age

42

LIE ABOUT YOUR AGE

In 1979, psychologist and Harvard professor Ellen Langer carried out a fascinating experiment with a group of men in their seventies and eighties, to explore the connection between mind and body.

Her mission: Find out whether if people dialed back their "age mind-set" a few decades, their body would follow.

Professor Langer did not tell the study's participants the true reason she was inviting them to a retreat. The men showed up believing they were simply there for a week of reminiscence.

As soon as the men arrived, they were sent on a time travel journey. Professor Langer surrounded the men with props, music, and films, all from the 1950s. She then asked the men to pretend it was 1959. They were encouraged to talk about Castro marching on Havana and the NASA satellite launch, all as if it were happening in the present. Professor Langer also removed any "aging prompts," like safety railings or walking sticks, that might make the men feel unhealthy.

Soon Professor Langer saw a big difference in the men. They were walking faster and behaving more confidently. By the end of the week one man even decided he no longer needed his walking stick.

Next up, Professor Langer rated the men's before and after physiology. She discovered a universal improvement in gait, dexterity, arthritis, physical speed, cognitive abilities, memory, blood pressure, vision, and hearing.

THE LESSON LEARNED: If you think of yourself as younger, you just might fool your body into thinking it's younger, too.

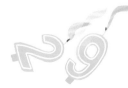

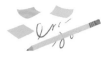

43

SCORE AN "A" AT HAVING A "C PERSONALITY"

Want to know a big secret to a longer life?

Nope—I'm not gonna tell you to cut back on skydiving. (Although people who follow this big secret might naturally tend not to be skydivers.)

The big secret: have a "C personality type"!

What does that mean? Researchers define C personality types as those who are *conscientious*—people who have a preference for planning, foresight, and caution.

There's a lot of research attesting to the life-powering perks of being a C personality—going as far back as a 1921 study on 1,500 children done by William Marston and Lewis Terman. Their data revealed one major commonality shared by their subjects who lived long into old age: conscientiousness.

Fast-forward to 2012—when researchers Howard Friedman and Leslie Martin took another look, in their famed book *The Longevity Project*. Once again, research supported that people who were conscientious enjoyed far greater longevity.

Researchers believe there are three major reasons why this quality leads to longer life:

1. **Conscientious people are slow and thoughtful decision makers.** They take time deciding on a marital partner, a career, or even what they're having for dinner. As a result, they find themselves in less stressful situations and enjoy far healthier partners and meals.

2. Conscientious folks are rule followers, which thereby protects health. For example, it can be very life-protective to wear a helmet while on a motorcycle!

3. Conscientious people tend to do research on risks. They are less prone to dangerous habits—like the aforementioned skydiving stuff—as well as risky habits like smoking cigarettes and enjoying frequent double cheeseburgers!

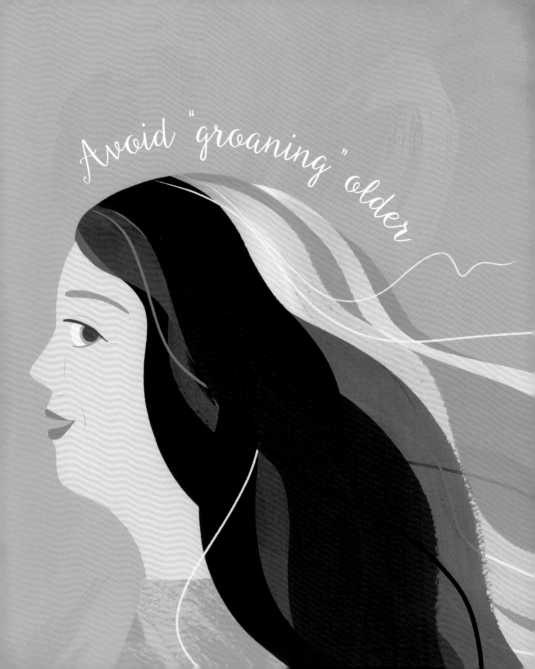

44

AVOID "GROANING" OLDER

Do you dread getting older?

Do you view each new gray hair as a red flag a-waving?

If so, you're not only hurting your daily mood, you're hurting your life span.

According to research from Becca R. Levy, PhD, and her associates at Yale University, adults with positive attitudes about aging lived more than seven years longer than their Negative Nelly peers.

According to these researchers, self-perceptions about aging had a greater impact on a person's life span than did the usual suspects: gender, socioeconomic status, loneliness levels, functional health, blood pressure, cholesterol, weight, or smoking status.

Basically, your self-perception about aging can become a self-fulfilling prophecy.

IT'S YOUR CHOICE:

1. Negative self-perceptions about aging = diminished life expectancy.

2. Positive self-perceptions about aging = prolonged life expectancy.

I'm picking choice #2!

45

YOU ARE WHO YOU EAT WITH

There's a familiar expression, "You are what you eat."

I've now created a new variation, which is equally true: "You are who you eat with!"

Basically, healthy living is contagious.

The scoop: According to Deakin University researchers, women who spend time around healthy peers were more likely to eat well and exercise.

The researchers believe there are a number of reasons why healthy habits can rub off on others.

The biggest reason: The desire to "fit in" with others is even more inspiring for developing healthy habits than the desire to fit into one's skinny jeans.

YOUR ASSIGNMENT: Purposefully find yourself a gang of "health buddies" who can serve as accountability buddies. Set the intention to lovingly create positive peer pressure with each other to eat healthier and work out more often.

BONUS: A report in the *British Medical Journal* suggests that people who exercise in a group burn an extra 500 calories a week compared to those who work out alone. Another example of "positive peer pressure" in action!

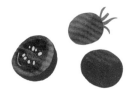

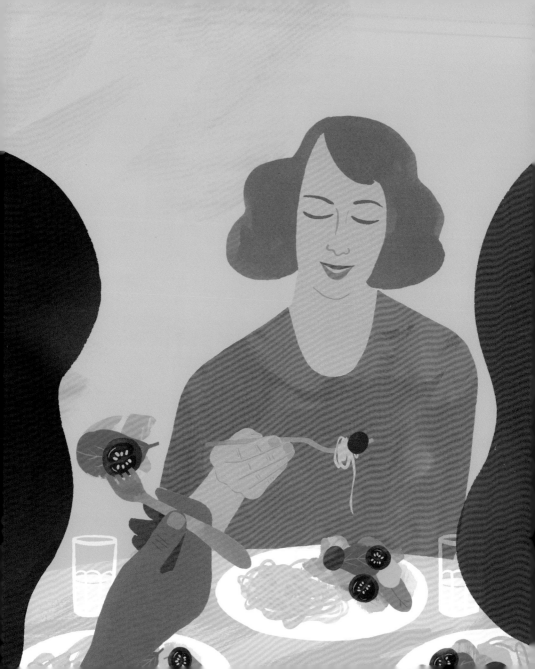

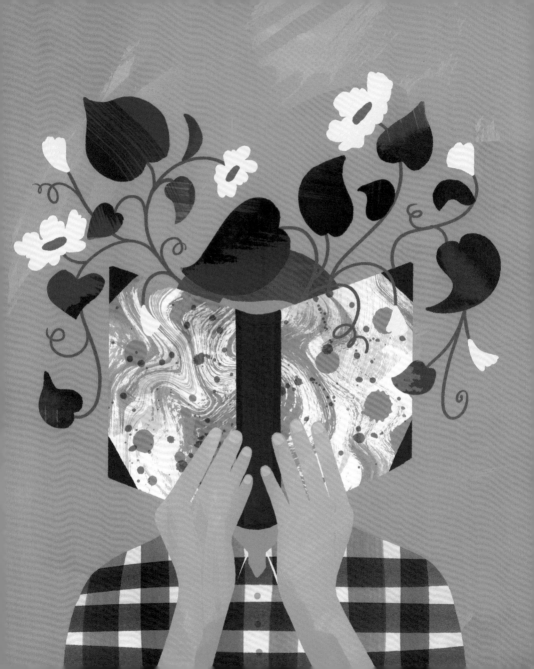

46

LIVE AND LEARN: THE MORE YOU LEARN, THE MORE YOU LIVE!

The National Institute on Aging found, in study after study, that the more you study, the longer you live.

Yep: getting a good long education ranked as the number one social factor for predicting whether you'll live a good long life—even more than the usual suspects like income and geographic region.

The math: Go to school for one extra year, boost your life expectancy one and a half years!

Hesitant to go to school because you think it's a waste of time? No worries. It's as if you'll get that time back!

Wondering why?

Theorists believe that people who love a good education are folks who also see the value in delaying gratification and planning for their future. These two qualities come in handy for staying alive.

After all, you need strong "delaying gratification muscles" if you're going to resist a jelly donut.

Plus, you need powerful "planning for the future muscles" if you're going to prioritize going to the gym rather than living for the moment and binge watching *Mad Men*.

Oh, and yes, you can strengthen your delaying gratification muscles.

WHAT TO DO? The more you do things like go to school and go to the gym, the easier it gets to want to delay gratification for your greater good—because you've witnessed the benefits of the greater good, and thereby have stronger motivation to wanna tap into your willpower for future challenges!

47

ILL FEELINGS CAN MAKE YOU ILL

There's a famous saying: "Anger is the poison you swallow hoping the other person dies." It turns out there's some truth to that.

The *Journal of the American College of Cardiology* reports that people who suffered from chronic anger were 19 percent more likely to develop heart problems than those who experienced anger less frequently.

Yelling is particularly bad for your health. "In the two hours after an angry outburst, the chance of having a heart attack doubles," says Chris Aiken, MD, director of the Mood Treatment Center in North Carolina.

Even recalling an angry experience can harm your health. Harvard University scientists asked healthy people to simply think about something that angered them, and these miffed memories caused a six-hour dip in levels of the antibody immunoglobulin A—the cells' first line of defense against infection.

If you try to repress your anger, that's not so healthy either. A University of Michigan study reported that couples who repress their anger experience shorter life spans than those who appropriately talk about their anger.

THE SOLUTION: Better communication skills and heaps of forgiveness.

Researchers, who titled their study report "Forgive to Live: Forgiveness, Health, and Longevity," found a link between unconditional forgiveness (not conditional forgiveness) and higher functioning cardiovascular, endocrine, and immune systems—and thereby lower mortality rates.

MY TIP TO FORGIVE AND LIVE:
Buy a huge bag of ice cubes.
Dump it all into your bathtub.
Tell yourself that by the time all
the ice melts down the drain,
you will release your
anger out of your
system.

Feelings

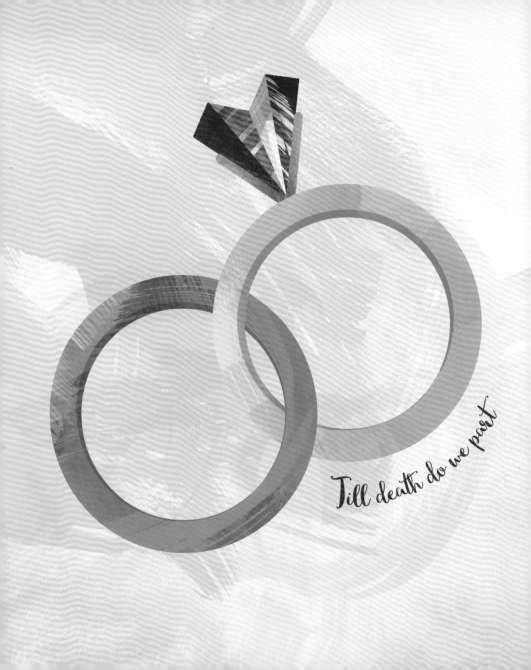

Till death do we part

48

PROMISING "TILL DEATH DO YOU PART" DELAYS WHEN YOU PART

Celebrity matchmaker Bonnie Winston loves to tell her clients that when she helps them get married she's simultaneously helping them live longer lives.

"There's a lot of research which supports that permanently partnered people are less likely to die early than single folks," says Ms. Winston. "There's a famous Duke University Medical Center study—plus a Harvard University Study as well."

Ms. Winston's right—and the studies go on and on!

Cardiologists at NYU's Langone Medical Center analyzed data from more than 3.5 million Americans and discovered married people age fifty and younger had a 12 percent less chance of developing any type of vascular disease than their unwed counterparts (independent of other cardiovascular risks). Plus, research found that men with wives were 46 percent less likely to die of heart disease than single guys (after taking into consideration diabetes, smoking, blood pressure, obesity, and other major risk factors).

Ms. Winston notes, "Of course, the health perks of marriage can be reversed if it's an unhappy relationship. If you want to kill each other, this constant stress can kill you off sooner!"

HER SOLUTION? "Be sure to marry someone you want to live with for a long time!"

49

BE THE RIGHT AMOUNT
OF POSITIVE

A 2012 aging study conducted by the Albert Einstein College of Medicine reported that enjoying optimism is a personality trait linked to longer life spans.

However, being a positive person doesn't necessarily increase your life on this planet.

In fact, your positivity could even be dangerous to your health!

Why?

According to researchers of the Longevity Project: "If you're . . . very optimistic, especially in the face of illness and recovery, if you don't consider the possibility that you might have setbacks, then those setbacks are harder to deal with—and could thereby lead to further health challenges."

IN SUMMARY: It helps to look on the bright side—but make sure all that brightness isn't blinding you from doing what you gotta do to wisely protect your health.

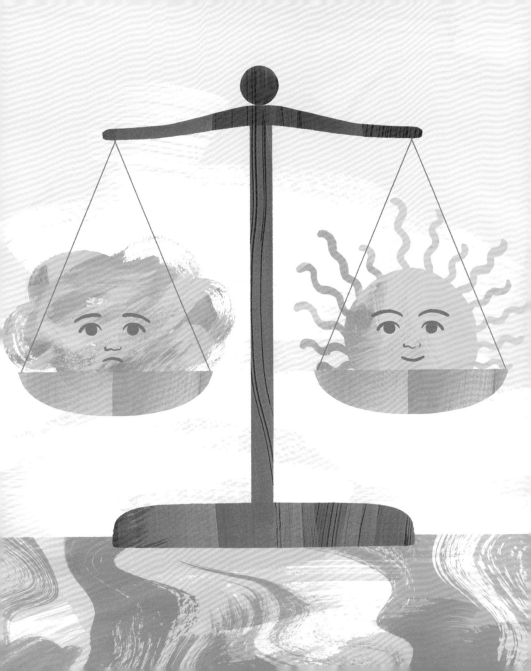

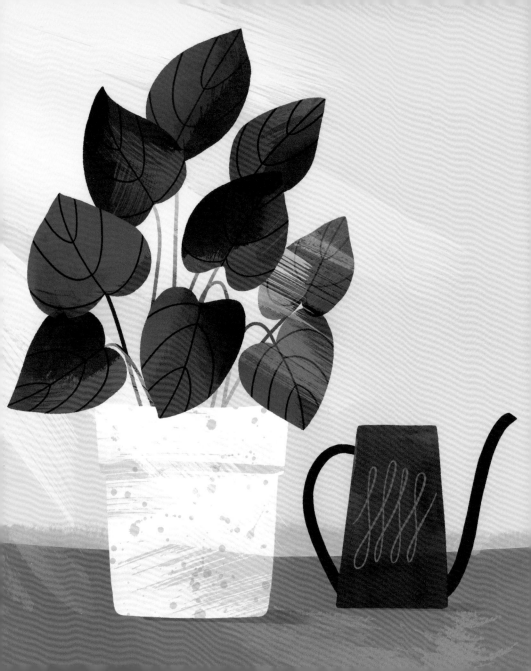

BE RESPONSIBLE FOR SOMETHING—EVEN A PLANT

If you want to keep growing older, you might want to grow a plant.

A fascinating study was performed on "plant keepers" in the 1970s by psychologists Judith Rodin and Ellen Langer. They split up residents in a Connecticut nursing home into two groups.

Group #1 was given a plant, plus the job of watering it. They were also invited to a lecture on the benefits of being responsible not only for the plant but also for their own lives.

Group #2 was also given a plant, but they were assigned someone else to water it. They were also invited to a lecture, but the topic was on how the staff was responsible for their well-being.

Fast-forward to a year and a half later:

Group #1 proved to be more active and alert than group #2. And fewer of the residents in group #1 had died.

THE LESSON LEARNED: When you take on responsibilities in your life, you can add on years to your life.

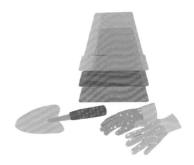

KEEP FAITHING FORWARD

It's already known: if you want to live longer, it's important to treat your body like a temple.

But you might not know that you can also live longer if you bring your body to an actual temple!

In WebMD's 2008 survey of centenarians, 84 percent say that staying in touch with their spirituality was "very important" for their healthy aging.

Researchers in a 2012 Nurses' Health Study found that women who went to church more than once a week had a 33 percent lower risk of dying during the study period, compared with those who never went.

Plus, 98 percent of the centenarians interviewed in the Blue Zones said they belonged to some type of faith-based community and held some form of a spiritual belief.

Meaning? The particular denomination of your spirituality doesn't matter.

Some researchers believe that the longevity perks that come from being religious are a by-product of joining a supportive community of fellow worshippers. But research also shows that you don't have to go to church, mosque, or synagogue to cash in on the longevity perks. You just have to have faith in a universal force that supports you during tough times.

The University of Maryland Medical Center notes, "Results from several studies indicate people with strong religious and spiritual beliefs heal faster from surgery, are less anxious and depressed, have lower blood pressure, and cope better with chronic illnesses," and that in a study of 232 heart surgery patients, religious folks were more likely to survive the first six months.

IN SUMMARY: If you want to delay heading off to heaven, it helps if you pray regularly to heaven—or simply maintain a spiritual practice of some kind, even if it's not a prayer-related one.

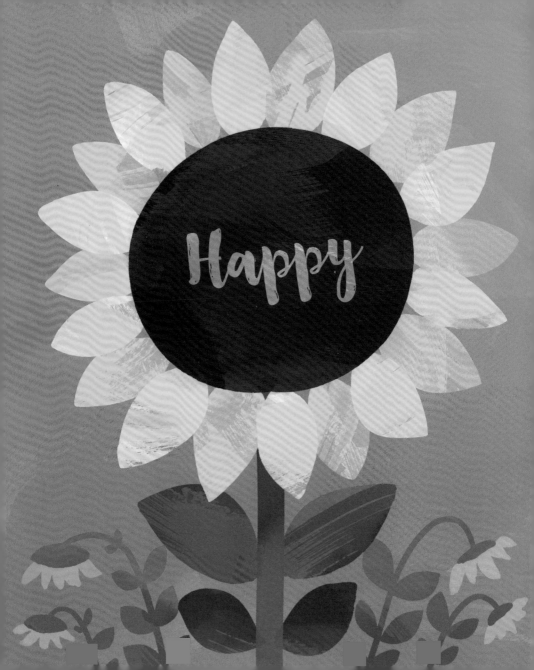

52

THE PERKIER YOUR MOOD, THE PERKIER YOUR BODY

Being happy boosts not only the quality of your life, but also the quantity of your life.

Here's the happily-and-healthier-ever-after research: Older people who reported feeling happy, excited, and/or content were up to 35 percent less likely to die during a five-year study conducted by the University College London. The study's researchers believe that positive emotions contribute to better health for two logical reasons:

- Brain regions connected to happiness are also involved in blood vessel function and inflammation.

- The stress hormone cortisol tends to rise and fall with emotions—the lower your cortisol levels, the better your health.

An American study also linked happiness with longer life. Professor Corey Keyes of Emory University reported that people who are "flourishing" (defined as "experiencing feelings of happiness and the ability to function smoothly in day-to-day life") are 60 percent less likely to die of premature causes. For this reason, Professor Keyes believes our health care system needs to include new psychological techniques to improve our moods as preventive measures.

TRANSLATION: One of the best antiaging tools is your brain. Master your thoughts to be positive, and you'll add more years to your life. Watch more funny movies, laugh more with friends, and spend more time on the hobbies and passions you love!

53

VANITY HELPS LONGEVITY

You know all that time you take to make sure your hair looks really good? (And it does!) Turns out, that's time well spent—because you can get that time back in the form of more years added onto your life.

Studies show that those who take time to look a little younger, live a little longer, says a report in *Perspectives on Psychological Science*, "The Influence of Age-Related Cues on Health and Longevity."

I know I always feel as if I have a little extra skip in my step after a good haircut. Now I know that I'm not imagining this result.

Here's the scoop: Women who think they look younger after having their hair colored and/or cut had a decrease in blood pressure. And they were also rated by others as younger looking in photos (although their hair was cropped out of the photo to eliminate that clue).

Basically, researchers believe that what you see youth-wise is what you get health-wise. External cues like youthful hair can affect how you age by influencing your health and life span.

IN SUMMARY: You now have lots of good health excuses to treat yourself to that chic new hairstyle. In fact, your life might just depend on it!

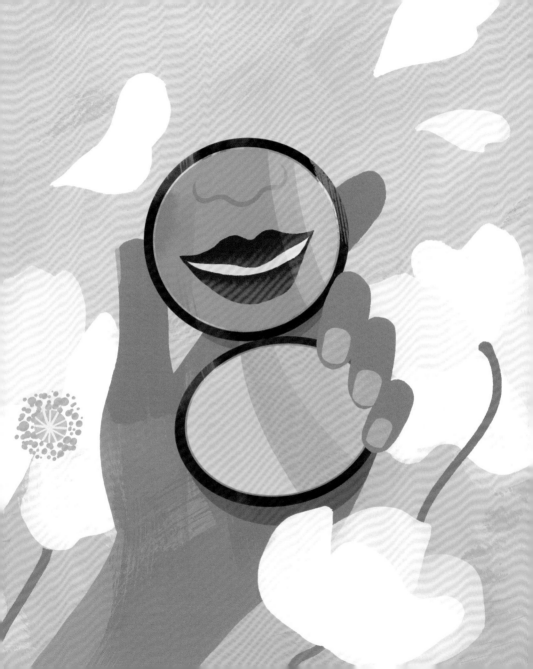

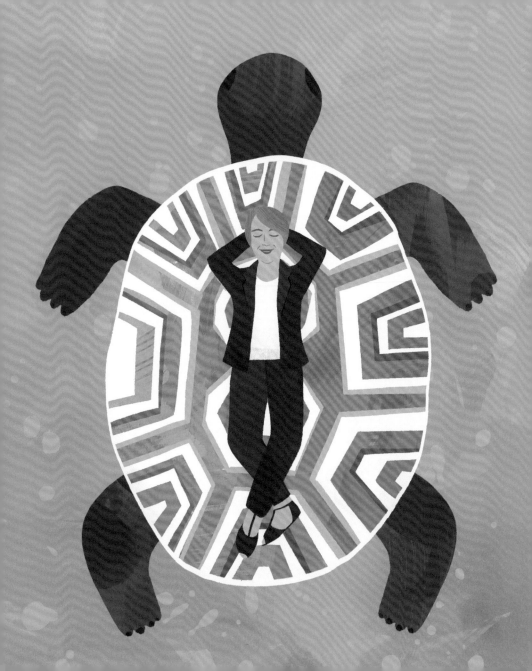

54

WARNING: BEING TOO CHILL CAN KILL!

You probably won't be too shocked to hear this: studies show that the more successful you are, the longer you live.

But you might be shocked to know this: you can die younger if you're too laid-back and carefree about work—and lack the motivation to succeed.

"There's a misconception about stress," says Dr. Howard S. Friedman, a University of California psychology professor who led a twenty-year study on aging. "People think everyone should take it easy." However, "a hard job that is also stressful can be associated with longevity."

Research by Annie Britton and Martin Shipley of University College London shows that if you're bored at work, you're twice as likely to suffer a heart attack or stroke over the next twenty-five years than folks who feel challenged and happy at work.

TWO REASONS WHY BEING TOO CHILL CAN KILL:

- Someone who is bored or not willing to work all that hard might also be someone who is less motivated to eat well, exercise, and all the rest of it.

- Someone who doesn't put passion into her work might also be depressed—and depression is a risk factor for heart disease.

IN SUMMARY: If you want to live a long and happy life, it's not enough to mildly want what you want. You must *wildly* want what you want. Don't shirk your work! Take on challenges!

55

FEELING GUILTY ABOUT NOT GOING TO THE GYM COULD BE BAD FOR YOUR HEALTH

Think you're not exercising as much as others? You need to improve your mind-set. Simply having guilt and insecurity about your fitness can be bad for your health!

In a study published in *Health Psychology*, Stanford University researchers Octavia Zahrt and Alia Crum discovered that participants who perceived themselves as less active than their friends tended to live shorter lives, even while exercising about as much.

In 2007, Crum studied hotel attendants who "were getting lots of exercise, but . . . didn't have the mind-set that their work was good exercise." Crum told some that their heavy lifting and walking *was* healthy exercise—and "the women who started to look at their work as good exercise had improvements in blood pressure and body fat."

Crum and Zahrt studied the physical activity, health, and personal backgrounds of over 61,000 American adults from three national health surveys, asking, "Compared with others your age, are you physically more active, less active, or equally active?" Then they viewed death records from twenty-one years, controlling for factors like physical activity, age, body mass index, and chronic illness.

Their conclusion: Individuals who believed they were less active than others were up to 71 percent more likely to die in the follow-up period than those who thought they were more active than their peers.

Shockingly, this mortality risk applied to people roughly similar to their peers— including their exercise levels! The researchers conjectured:

- Those who *believed* they were getting enough exercise wound up experiencing greater physiological benefits. Conversely, an underlying fear of not exercising could undermine health.

- Perceptions affected motivation. Zahrt explains, "People who think they are less active can be discouraged by that perception, and they might stop exercising and become less active." This might have led to some of the negative health outcomes— although Zahrt tried to control for exercise similarities.

YOUR ASSIGNMENT: Don't compare or scare yourself to exercise; *inspire* yourself with a positive mind-set.

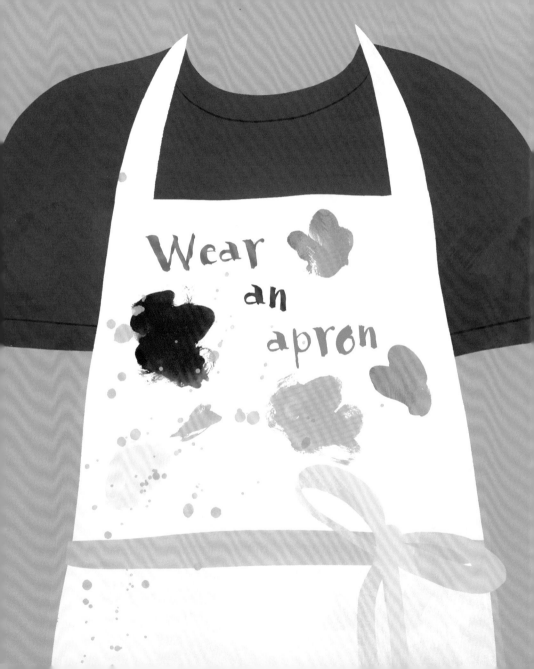

56

WEAR AN APRON

If you're presently using your oven to store old sweaters, you might want to rethink that!

It turns out that making good old-fashioned home-cooked meals can help you live to a good old age.

A 2012 study of elderly Taiwanese reported in *Public Health Nutrition* found that those who cooked up to five times a week had a 47 percent greater chance of staying alive over a ten-year period.

The reasons vary:

- You're more in control of the ingredients.
- You're more active in mind and body—thinking up meals and shopping for ingredients.

"It has become clear that cooking is a healthy behavior," said Professor Mark Wahlqvist, the lead author of the study. "It deserves a place in lifelong education, public health policy, urban planning, and household economics."

REMINDER: Don't be a kook about what and how you cook! Make sure you're cooking healthfully, with the right kinds of oils, and not too much salt or sugar.

57

SMILE BIGGER

Here's a quirky fact, which will not only make you smile but also inspire you to smile *bigger*. The actual size of your smile might make a difference in how long you live.

In a 2009 study published in *Psychological Science*, researchers examined the intensity of smiles in photos of baseball players from the 1950s, since deceased.

The players with no smile in their picture had lived, on average, 72.9 years.

The biggest smilers had lived, on average, 79.9 years—a whopping seven years longer!

EXTRA REASON TO SMILE: You just finished reading this entire book, which means you're loaded up with info to live longer and younger! Plus, since you've read all the way to the last page, this shows you're blessed with the trait of conscientiousness—which (as mentioned in #43: Score an "A" at Having a "C Personality") increases your longevity potential. Yay you!

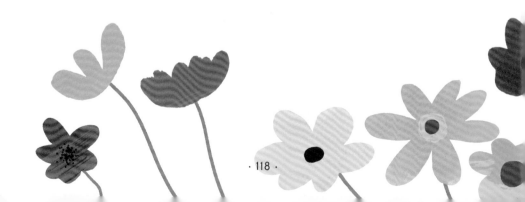

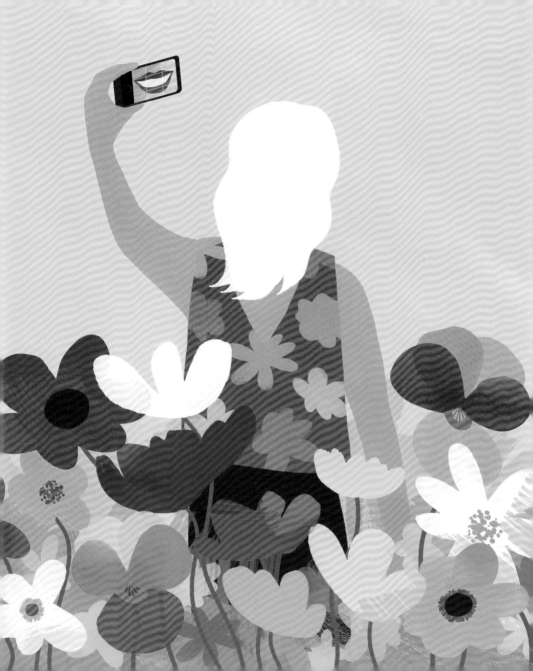

Index

I'd like to dedicate this book to both my son, Ari Salmansohn, and my mom, Gloria Salmansohn.

Thank you, Mom, for being such an inspiring role model for aging gracefully, energetically, and gorgeously. Each day you give me reason to believe I can live longer and younger.

Thank you, my amazing son Ari, for inspiring this book—and giving me infinite reasons to want to live as close to forever as I can!

Copyright © 2018 by Karen Salmansohn
Illustrations copyright © 2018 by Sarah Ferone

All rights reserved.
Published in the United States by Ten Speed Press, an imprint of the Crown Publishing Group, a division of Penguin Random House LLC, New York.
www.crownpublishing.com
www.tenspeed.com

Ten Speed Press and the Ten Speed Press colophon are registered trademarks of Penguin Random House LLC.

Library of Congress Cataloging-in-Publication Data

Names: Salmansohn, Karen, author.
Title: Life is long : 50+ ways to help you live a little bit closer to
   forever / Karen Salmansohn, best-selling author of Think Happy.
Description: First edition. | New York : Ten Speed Press, [2018] | Includes
   bibliographical references and index.
Identifiers: LCCN 2017050280 | ISBN 9780399580703 (hardcover) | ISBN
   9780399580710 (ebook)
Subjects: LCSH: Longevity. | Self-care, Health.
Classification: LCC RA776.75 .S24 2018 | DDC 613.2—dc23
LC record available at https://lccn.loc.gov/2017050280

Hardcover ISBN: 978-0-399-58070-3
eBook ISBN: 978-0-399-58071-0

Printed in China

Design by Leona Chelsea Legarte

10 9 8 7 6 5 4 3 2 1

First Edition